SAVING

the Art of

MEDICINE

Observations of a Practitioner

ALLEN SUSSMAN MD

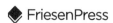 FriesenPress

One Printers Way
Altona, MB R0G 0B0
Canada

www.friesenpress.com

ISBN
978-1-03-916179-5 (Hardcover)
978-1-03-916178-8 (Paperback)
978-1-03-916180-1 (eBook)

1. Medical, Physician & Patient

Distributed to the trade by The Ingram Book Company

SAVING
the Art of
MEDICINE

SAVING
the Art of
MEDICINE

To my soulmate and late wife
Melanie

who taught me so much about life

TABLE OF CONTENTS

PREFACE

Fifty years of practice and contemplation taught me that medicine is both an art and a science. Unfortunately, we have glorified the science in modern healthcare while losing sight of the art. I hope to offer a unique overview of the field, one that is wide-ranging and theoretical, even as it is grounded in the practical details of my day-to-day encounters with patients.

As a practicing endocrinologist, actively engaged in the study of cholesterol, hypertension, diabetes, and osteoporosis, I gained tremendous insight into the advantages and drawbacks of evidence-based medicine. Currently, the dominance of the clinical trial, as well as other trends such as the commodification of healthcare and the rapid influx of new technologies, is causing doctors to lose sight of the essence of their practice—connecting with their patients as individual human beings.

Working to resolve my patients' health issues, often over the course of many years, I grew to appreciate the extraordinary significance of our personal interactions. I went from being bookish to mindful to heartfelt. I learned that being a doctor is about so much more than applying the science taught in medical school. It is about cultivating one's humanity, a lifelong process that is intensely personal. Medicine is not just the implementation of scientific precepts and the administration of drugs. It is, above all, a profound process of connecting the part with the whole.

In describing my journey, I've wanted to convey that the practice of medicine is essentially multi-faceted and that we ignore this truth at our peril. The result is a book that does not fit nicely into any one genre. Some readers may be drawn to the stories of human inter-relationship, while others will enjoy the scientific analysis of medical practice. Still others will appreciate discussions that highlight the uncertainties that pervade the medical field or allude to that which remains mysterious because it cannot be perceived by the senses. Perhaps your credulity will be strained as I discuss esoteric phenomena, but you still value a holistic approach that integrates personal observation and intuition. No matter your perspective or inclinations, hopefully your understanding of the field will be expanded in some new direction that will be of benefit to you either as a provider of healthcare or receiver. Consider this book a kaleidoscope that reveals various patterns; you get to choose where you linger, absorbing the new colors and shapes.

Ultimately, I do not advocate a specific spiritual approach or healing modality but believe in freeing ourselves from dogma and learning all that we can from the various approaches available to us, from allopathic to alternative. What my journey taught me and what I hope it may convey to readers, whether or not they work in the field, is that the best healthcare is rooted in an intimate understanding of the larger picture, one that is ultimately mysterious and awe-inspiring.

In high school, I had to write a short story. I had no idea what to do and was racked with anxiety. In the end, I chose to describe a man who gets shipwrecked on an island and lives in solitude for the rest of his life. He gains a good deal of knowledge about how to survive and, having accepted that he'll never interact with another human being again, decides to write down some of the wisdom he has gained. A volcanic explosion occurs, causing major earthquakes, and the land begins to sink into the ocean. The man puts his papers into a bottle and caps it just before the island is completely flooded and he himself disappears. All that is left is the bottle containing the thoughts and ideas he has accumulated over the years, bobbing in the vast, watery expanse.

PREFACE

Fifty years of practice and contemplation taught me that medicine is both an art and a science. Unfortunately, we have glorified the science in modern healthcare while losing sight of the art. I hope to offer a unique overview of the field, one that is wide-ranging and theoretical, even as it is grounded in the practical details of my day-to-day encounters with patients.

As a practicing endocrinologist, actively engaged in the study of cholesterol, hypertension, diabetes, and osteoporosis, I gained tremendous insight into the advantages and drawbacks of evidence-based medicine. Currently, the dominance of the clinical trial, as well as other trends such as the commodification of healthcare and the rapid influx of new technologies, is causing doctors to lose sight of the essence of their practice—connecting with their patients as individual human beings.

Working to resolve my patients' health issues, often over the course of many years, I grew to appreciate the extraordinary significance of our personal interactions. I went from being bookish to mindful to heartfelt. I learned that being a doctor is about so much more than applying the science taught in medical school. It is about cultivating one's humanity, a lifelong process that is intensely personal. Medicine is not just the implementation of scientific precepts and the administration of drugs. It is, above all, a profound process of connecting the part with the whole.

In describing my journey, I've wanted to convey that the practice of medicine is essentially multi-faceted and that we ignore this truth at our peril. The result is a book that does not fit nicely into any one genre. Some readers may be drawn to the stories of human inter-relationship, while others will enjoy the scientific analysis of medical practice. Still others will appreciate discussions that highlight the uncertainties that pervade the medical field or allude to that which remains mysterious because it cannot be perceived by the senses. Perhaps your credulity will be strained as I discuss esoteric phenom-ena, but you still value a holistic approach that integrates personal observation and intuition. No matter your perspective or inclinations, hopefully your understanding of the field will be expanded in some new direction that will be of benefit to you either as a provider of healthcare or receiver. Consider this book a kaleidoscope that reveals various patterns; you get to choose where you linger, absorbing the new colors and shapes.

Ultimately, I do not advocate a specific spiritual approach or healing modality but believe in freeing ourselves from dogma and learning all that we can from the various approaches available to us, from allopathic to alternative. What my journey taught me and what I hope it may convey to readers, whether or not they work in the field, is that the best healthcare is rooted in an intimate understanding of the larger picture, one that is ultimately mysterious and awe-inspiring.

In high school, I had to write a short story. I had no idea what to do and was racked with anxiety. In the end, I chose to describe a man who gets shipwrecked on an island and lives in solitude for the rest of his life. He gains a good deal of knowledge about how to survive and, having accepted that he'll never interact with another human being again, decides to write down some of the wisdom he has gained. A volcanic explosion occurs, causing major earthquakes, and the land begins to sink into the ocean. The man puts his papers into a bottle and caps it just before the island is completely flooded and he himself disappears. All that is left is the bottle containing the thoughts and ideas he has accumulated over the years, bobbing in the vast, watery expanse.

GROUNDWORK

"There are more things in heaven and earth, Horatio, than are dreamt of in your philosophy."

William Shakespeare, *Hamlet*

CHAPTER ONE

The Art of Medicine

Medicine is rushing full throttle into the technological and informational age. At the beginning of my practice, X-rays were the main means of imaging, but now CAT scans and MRIs have become commonplace. Limb prosthetics have been developed that can be controlled by the mind. And artificial intelligence is assisting doctors in a number of areas, from clinical decision-making to performing surgery. In many ways, the role of the doctor seems to be shrinking. In contrast, for most of history, healthcare was defined by the relationship between patient and healer. There was no "evidence-based" medicine using the scientific method. Market forces and profit were not the drivers of change.

Are we better off for the change? The answer is yes and no. Everyone appears to want the latest technology and treatment options. On the other hand, many patients are disillusioned with the medical system because of the lack of personal interaction and compassion. The new buzzword in the corporate mega-healthcare system is "patient-based" medicine, but it has quickly become another glib term bandied about while the autonomy of the patient and the role of the doctor are diminished. The system declares that the patient is the star, but rules, arbitrary and inhuman, are quick to tell you otherwise. The philosopher Ivan Illich, portending the current medical crisis, saw modern medicine as "an engineering endeavor" built on the belief that good health is "the result of technical manipulation." He went so far as to say it had turned into "a sick-making enterprise" (Illich, 2016, p.98).

Even as I was immersed in the day-to-day practice of medicine, I realized that there was a story to be told of my growing understanding of the medical profession. Often, it was my patients who taught and guided me. The process was dynamic and constantly evolving, with countless emotional highs and lows along the way. I changed in ways that were sometimes so slow and profound, I would not realize it till years later.

What I learned is that facts pertaining to the purely physical realm present only a partial truth. In fact, there is no purely physical realm. There is mind and body, spiritual and physical interconnected. And there is the interconnection between ourselves and the truth, bringing into play faith, belief, and art. As a student, I was steeped in science, and as a practicing physician, I felt a profound respect for the value of scientific endeavor. At the same time, I have learned that science is a belief like any other and has its biases. We can never know the truth separate from our knowing of it. This can be lamented or celebrated since it speaks to the interconnectedness of all things and how we are an inseparable part of the whole. Instead of pursuing the illusion of objective truth, we can open ourselves to the mystery of life and support each other as events unfold. Doctors who have the humility and open-mindedness to orient themselves in this way are practicing the art, and not just the science, of medicine.

A HISTORICAL VIEW

When I started medical school, I knew nothing of the history of medicine and assumed that the practice of medicine was one of continual development, a constant accumulation of facts using ever more sophisticated analyses. An overview of the last three millennia of medical practice, focusing on the West, does give us a picture of radical transformation; at the same time, important areas of ancient wisdom and practice have been relegated to insignificance. Let us explore the past to understand the present path of medicine—what has been lost along the way, as well as gained.

The first healers may well have been the shamans that lived in the Neolithic era. In modern times, shamanism is practiced in select communities and has at its heart the close relationship between healer and patient. The intimacy of this therapeutic relationship is essential to the success of any treatments, and it is via ritual that the healer accesses the spiritual realm in order to gain insight into a person's physical condition, something that is hard to understand from a scientific perspective. Herbal products found in nature are administered but only as part of an unfolding interaction. Perhaps the placebo effect is at work, as we will discuss later. Perhaps trance states with energetic potential promote healing. These are realms that modern medicine shies away from.

The beginnings of modern medicine can be traced back to Greece, Hippocrates being the preeminent figure. He is considered the father of modern medicine, and medical schools still have their students recite the Hippocratic Oath at graduation, with the most important message being *Primum non nocere*: First, do no harm. Hippocratic medicine was the collaborative outcome of several centuries of accumulating wisdom about the body. The supernatural systems that had been used to account for disease as an expression of the wrath of deities were supplanted by observation of the patient. Objective measures began to be used, such as taking a pulse.

Even so, the system was largely philosophical, as opposed to experimental. The body's dysfunction was understood as an imbalance of the four humors— blood, yellow bile, black bile, and phlegm. The excesses were corrected by the use of purgatives, emetics, bloodletting, and sweating. While these methods would in modern times be considered dubious, the practice in general was characterized by high moral and ethical standards. "With purity and holiness, I will pass my life and practice my art." These are words from the Hippocratic Oath. A beautiful precept was: "Where there is a love of humankind, there is also a love of the art of medicine."

Hippocrates established a system of precepts and observations to be passed on to other practitioners. The overall approach was to let the patient heal naturally without inflicting harm but instead supporting the body via diet, rest, and reassurance. Many wise words can be found among these sayings. Consider the first aphorism: "Life is short, and art long; the crisis fleeting; experience perilous, and decision difficult."

The system remained dogma through most of the Middle Ages, with the most significant contributions coming from Galen in the second century AD. He designed a more coherent system of looking at the four humors and promoted the idea of an inherent vitalism that is predetermined and ordained. Complex herbal concoctions were developed and remained in use for over a millennium. Anatomical and physiological investigations were performed—on animals since human dissection was not allowed for moral reasons. The results were thought to reveal the predetermined plans of the demiurge, the figure in Platonic philosophy who was responsible for shaping the material universe. Still, the experimentation showed the beginnings of a scientific impulse. While many of the theoretical concepts were later debunked, it was an attempt at a reasoned approach, and it was preserved during the Middle Ages, in part thanks to physicians from the Middle East like Avicenna. His *Canon of Medicine*, completed in the eleventh century, incorporated the Hippocratic and Galen legacies as well as Arabic practices and allowed for a codification of medical practices that would otherwise have been lost.

During this same period, gifted healers in Europe promoted a holistic approach to healing. In the twelfth century, Hildegard of Bingen, a polymath with interests in music, theology, and herbology, grew her own herbs and was extremely knowledgeable regarding their use. Her overall approach towards illness was to give time and nature a chance to effect a positive result. Victoria Sweet in *God's Hotel* describes how she used Hildegard's precepts of "slow" medicine to help the chronically sick and disadvantaged people in a twentieth-century almshouse. It's an approach that has been lost in our fast-paced, results-driven, modern medical system.

The first big movements towards modern medical understanding occurred in the sixteenth century. The medieval Church had curtailed certain avenues of exploration, but during the Renaissance, people began to pursue knowledge outside of a religious context, eagerly investigating physical phenomena as well as the powers of technology. Later, during the Age of Reason, mainstream Western culture and society progressed further along this path, away from spiritual approaches to understanding. The world was becoming steadily objectified and rationalized. Major advancements in our knowledge of the body were made, accompanied by losses in our more spiritual sensibilities.

In the Renaissance, Paracelsus developed an approach that was grounded in observable phenomena but that remained spiritual. Practicing in the first half of the sixteenth century, he was one of the first to insist that physicians be trained in the natural sciences, in particular chemistry. He replaced the prevailing theory of the four humors with a system of three chemicals, sulfur, salt, and mercury, representing the principles of flammability, solidity, and volatility. Disease was connected to local causes that came from a vital force with a spiritual resonance. He was reworking the old concepts and trying to develop a more physiological system that still maintained an aura of otherworldliness. He turned to nature for treatment options. He believed that "nature was illegible to proud professors, but clear to pious adepts" (Porter, 1997, p.202). Observation and experimentation became more important than traditional dogma. At the same time, Paracelsus would follow a doctrine of signatures that was hard to understand. For example, since the plant eyebright resembled a blue eye, it was to be used in eye ailments. His views were clearly not evolved by modern standards. Nonetheless, his reverence for nature has had a strong influence on present-day alternative medicine practice.

The Enlightenment saw dramatic scientific advances, putting an end to both the four-humor paradigm and the chemical Paracelsian model. Of critical importance were Harvey's advances in the field of experimental physiology, above all the discovery in 1628 of the blood circulation system. Also, Harvey effectively launched the field of quantitative measurements when he calculated how much blood was pumped out of the heart. He reasoned that, since this amount could not be continually produced and dissipated, it was being preserved and recirculated. This dramatic advance in our understanding of the body's organization would spur more discoveries regarding the cardiopulmonary system and oxygenation.

Another British subject of the seventeenth century, Thomas Sydenham, posthumously given the moniker of the English Hippocrates, advanced the practice of medicine by promoting a bedside manner as well as the use of direct observation to diagnose a disorder without reliance on pathological anatomy or microscopic analysis. There are many marvelous quotes ascribed to him, including: "I have consulted my patients' safety and my own reputation most effectually by doing nothing at all."

Of tremendous significance for the advance of medicine as a healing art was the connection made between the knowledge of anatomy and the study of individual cases and conditions. This began in the 1500s, by which point the dissection of human cadavers had become acceptable, and Vesalius, with the dissection skills of a genius, published his opus *On the Structure of the Human Body*. Two centuries later, Morgagni, building on Vesalius's work, established anatomy as the instrument to identify disease by showing the practical consequences of a scientific understanding of structure. He correlated seven hundred detailed case reports with the pathologic anatomical findings in a coherent indexed fashion, so physicians could use the information in their decision-making.

It was also during the Enlightenment that the first reputed clinical trial took place, performed by James Lind in 1747. The idea of setting up an experiment to compare the outcomes for separately defined groups began with a study that was quaint by modern standards, each group containing just one pair of sailors. The twelve sailors in total had been at sea for two months and were showing signs of scurvy. Their diet was the same, but one of every pair was given an additional daily substance—cider, elixir of vitriol (sulfuric acid), vinegar, seawater, oranges and lemon, or barley water. After six days, the trial was stopped because there was no more fruit available. Of the pair given fruit, they had either totally or partially recovered. Otherwise, only the cider group showed some improvement. It was not a very sophisticated study and in no shape or form passes the minimum criteria for a randomized clinical trial. There was no randomization, nor a well-developed, systematic plan. But it was a significant precursor.

As scientific experimentation advanced, certain aspects of medicine suffered. By the eighteenth century, physicians were becoming part of a trade. They had developed an objective clinical gaze and a paternalistic attitude. While in the past, family, neighbors, and priests had been active in allaying suffering and promoting healing, now it was only examination by the medical professional that counted. Even the patient's own description of symptoms was considered irrelevant, too subjective compared to the results of a clinical, physical examination. Voltaire ridiculed this state of affairs: "Doctors are men who prescribe medicines of which they know little, to cure diseases of which they know less, in human beings of whom they know nothing."

Nonetheless, science, in its inexorable, plodding way, made dramatic discoveries, leading to a dramatic expansion of the armamentarium of helpful agents over the next two hundred years. Often, scientists learned about the world without immediately knowing the practical benefits, paving the way for medical breakthroughs later. As Isaac Newton explained in a letter to his fellow scientist Robert Hooke in 1675, "If I have seen further, it is by standing on the shoulders of giants." Science is a team game without instant gratification.

The field of infectious disease is a stellar example of this gradual, cumulative process. First, on the technological front, a steady evolution allowed for examinations of the body beyond our gross visual perceptions. In the mid-seventeenth century, the microscope, developed by Leeuwenhoek, gave us our first view of the micro world. Two centuries later, the Zeiss workshop produced the compound microscope, allowing for vastly more detailed examinations. At that time, the first liquid artificial culture medium was created by Louis Pasteur, and staining was discovered as a useful way to better identify microbes.

Meanwhile, as tools of observation grew more sophisticated, creating a wealth of data regarding the microscopic world, there were crucial developments in theory. Here, too, we can observe a clear progression. The use of the word "cell" to describe the basic unit of life was first used by Robert Hooke in the seventeenth century. Two centuries later, Virchow, building on cell theory, stressed that most of the diseases of mankind could be understood in terms of dysfunction on a cellular level, not on the level of gross anatomy. Around the same time, Pasteur's germ theory proved that bacteria are the cause of disease, not miasma from rotting material. Procedures were sought to zero in on the culprits, and at the end of the nineteenth century, a narrow set of criteria, known as Koch's postulates, was developed to establish whether a particular organism is the cause of a particular disease. The microorganism must: 1) be present in all disease cases, 2) isolated and grown in a pure culture, 3) inoculated into a healthy lab animal who then develops the disease, and 4) re-isolated. In 1928, Alexander Fleming found a green mold contaminating his microbial culture and killing the bacteria. Antibiotics were developed soon after: first synthetic antibiotics in 1935, with the production of the sulfa drug Protonsil from a commercial dye, and then in 1942, penicillin, created from the mold that Fleming discovered.

Another extraordinary illustration of the process of scientific advance has been the development of vaccines, starting with the work of eighteenth-century pioneer Edward Jenner, who gets credit for the first smallpox vaccine—inoculating cowpox—that was already well-known to dairy maids. Pasteur in 1885 created an attenuated strain of the rabies virus to serve as a vaccine, and this in turn paved the way for vaccines for tuberculosis, diphtheria, and tetanus in the pre-antibiotic era of the 1920's. Note that the first agents to control infections were vaccines, not antibiotics, and that their use predates scientific examination.

As doctors' and scientists' insight into disease and its treatment grew, previous theories and practices were debunked. One such practice was bloodletting, which had been prescribed for centuries for a host of problems. In 1835, Pierre Louis conducted a trial to determine the efficacy of bloodletting as a treatment for pneumonia. He discovered that it did not change the course of the illness in toto. In fact, while certain patients did recover faster, there was overall an increase in mortality. One can only wonder what would have happened to George Washington just a few decades earlier if he'd been spared the multiple phlebotomies to which he was subjected upon developing an upper respiratory infection. The general opinion is that he would have survived if he'd been spared treatment.

In general, old concepts of ethereal substances with philosophical meaning were gradually replaced by a more and more detailed picture of the physiology of the body. In 1865, Claude Bernard, while exploring such phenomena as pancreatic juices and liver glycogenesis, created the concept of "milieu interieur," to refer to an internal environment that remains stable despite a changing outside world. He became the founder of modern physiology, replacing the ancient idea of life forces with a mechanistic process of regulation. In 1926, Walter Cannon, head of physiology at Harvard, built on Bernard's concept, coining the term "homeostasis" to describe the dynamic system of regulation that maintains the stability of the internal milieu by keeping a multitude of specific variables within an extremely narrow range. Life could be seen as a high-wire balancing act, governed by the continual need to respond to perturbations caused by external stimuli. Chemical laboratory testing became an increasingly important part of the medical exam, with lab ranges dictating the normal variance of substances in the blood and anything outside that range becoming a cause for concern.

Building on the work of the past few centuries, our current era is marked by the standardization of both medical care and scientific investigation. A critical threshold was crossed with the release in 1910 of the Flexner Report, under the aegis of the Carnegie Foundation, authored by a man with an academic, not medical, background. It presented an approach to medical training that was based on the German model and designed to promote the best medical teaching practices found at Johns Hopkins. Rigid standards were promulgated to strengthen the scientific basis of medicine. Medical schools would be conducting research while physicians would be hired to teach, paid by the institution and not by the patient.

William Osler voiced his concerns over the lack of attention to clinical care, calling the report "a very good thing for science, but a very bad thing for the profession" (Starr, 2017, p.122-123). A professor at Johns Hopkins and the first to bring medical students out of the lecture hall for bedside clinical training, he felt the report diminished the all-important relationship between patient and doctor. The report was also a death knell to many schools of naturopathy and homeopathy and proprietary schools for profit.

Standards were put in place for the field of investigation as well. In 1948, the first randomized clinical trial (RCT) took place, spawning a profusion of studies and prompting the need for standardization of practice and assessment. Canadian epidemiologist David Sackett responded by rating the studies according to a rigorously defined set of criteria. As one of the pioneers of "evidence-based medicine," he ensured that the RCT became the primary avenue of scientific investigation. Between 1969 and 2018, over 175,000 RCTs of varying quality have been published. Citations of these papers number over six million.

RCTs, and the metanalyses and guidelines they spawn, have become the bread and butter of medical teaching institutions and Big Pharma. Each party has its own agenda, with medical schools gaining stature and recognition for their medical prowess, and Big Pharma promoting sales and enlarging their market share. The focus has shifted from infectious diseases to chronic, complicated disorders and their "cures." Economics plays an increasingly dominant role, as multiple parties fight over finances—patients, provider, insurance companies, Big Pharma, and the government.

In some ways, the alienation that began in the Enlightenment and continued through the Industrial Age has become more pronounced. "The sick person has become a thing," said the German physician Robert Volz in the 1800s, and that critique is still relevant today (Porter, 1997, p.311). Evidence and standardization have been glorified at the expense of the individual human being. We live in a

Mechanical Age, of which Thomas Carlyle said, "nothing is now done directly, or by hand; all is by rule and calculated contrivance" (Carlyle, 2001, p.34).

Still, today's respected clinicians are made from the same cloth as Thomas Sydenham back in the seventeenth century. Humility and connection to the patient is clearly an ageless quality among physicians. It is my fervent belief that we need to reaffirm these basic values. As we have seen, the field of medicine has evolved dramatically over time. Scientific progress has been astounding. At the same time, an over-emphasis on the gathering of facts has led to the objectification of medical problems, and the human relationship between patient and doctor has suffered. A historical overview reveals that the practice of medicine is a constantly evolving phenomenon. It shows us where we have been and where we are now. This gives us all the more power and freedom to change course and craft new visions for the future.

CHAPTER TWO

Training and Early Practice

When I first decided to become a doctor, I was enthralled by the scientific process of discovery, but even more than that, I longed for direct interaction with people, wanting both to learn from them and help them. My father was a family doctor practicing in the Bronx, and I was impressed with the respect and love his patients had for him. He worked seven days a week and made house calls as well. Health insurance was not the norm, and my dad often accepted gifts in lieu of cash. In this way, he acquired oil paintings by accomplished artists as well as signed copies of a book by Chaim Potok, a well-known Yiddish author. In the beginning, his visits took him after hours to distressed areas, but after his car was stolen twice, he stopped that practice. Once, when he was up late in his small office, a drug addict held him up at knife point. Still, his dedication to his patients did not waver. He was the doctor I wanted to become.

A MEDICAL EDUCATION

Following in my father's footsteps, I did not seek the high compensation of a medical specialty. I was above all interested in the human mind, and New York Medical College, with a progressive and well-known psychiatric staff, seemed a good fit. I soon changed my focus, however. During electives, I found myself in a clinic serving Latina teenagers whose mothers, fearful that their daughters would be assaulted or defiled, did not allow them out of their apartments, and they became socially and psychologically deprived. I felt completely powerless to help them, nor did I see a ray of hope coming from the skilled psychiatric staff.

I pivoted to endocrinology, hoping to immerse myself in the study of mind-body connections. Scientific study is essential to becoming a proficient endocrinologist, whose decision-making is based on well-executed experiments and clinical trials, but the appeal of this particular specialty was its breadth, the study of all the organ systems, unlike the specialties of cardiology, gastroenterology, or nephrology, which treat specific organs, mostly in isolation. Hormones are the focus, and the prospect of putting together a puzzle with multiple pieces, both physical and psycho-emotional, was exciting to me. It seemed the most holistic practice I could aspire to. Moreover, the field would allow for a good deal of personal contact with patients.

My early training, however, completely deemphasized patients and their humanity and in no way promoted a holistic approach. I had to do a lot of studying in the first two years to become fluent in Medicalese, and I came to believe that this gauntlet of rigorous, strategically planned courses would mold me into a competent healer. The sheer number of facts to be learned left no time for the beauty and art of medical care. Compassion for the patients was low on my list of priorities.

I was taught that good medicine meant understanding the facts and delivering them. And certainly, learning about the workings of the body was fascinating. I enjoyed the courses in physiology and biochemistry as well as anatomy, the quintessential course in all medical schools. Our bible was *Gray's Anatomy*. Then there was the work of Frank Netter, who raised anatomical renditions to an art form. "A picture is worth a thousand words" is particularly apt where his drawings are concerned.

The first time I went beyond book-learning, it was not to meet with a patient but with a cadaver. Gross anatomy could indeed be gross, depending on the condition of the corpse. Since medical school started in the fall, bodies were collected over the summer, and that year, there happened to be a prolonged blackout in New York City. The freezers were affected, and our very first day, we had to practice amputation—to eliminate the decomposing tissue that was infested with maggots. Needless to say, that experience did not motivate me to become a surgeon. We tried to relate to the corpse by giving it a name, but in retrospect, I believe we did it out of a macabre sense of humor as well as acute feelings of discomfort at finding ourselves in the presence of an inert, unfeeling corpse.

Eventually, I did meet with a live patient, but the experience was hardly meaningful. I was assigned to see a patient in his hospital room, without the benefit of being introduced by another physician. I had been studying *Bedside Diagnostic Examination* by DeGowin and DeGowin, zeroing in on the section about the abdomen, since I was told the patient had liver cancer. We had been given some handouts and lectures on getting a history from the patient, including details of social and family history. I was supposed to practice a prescribed way of addressing and examining a patient. The rigidity of the protocol was meant to decrease the risk of missing important information. There was so much information to gather that there was no time to develop any kind of connection with the patient. In fact, all that I remember about this patient is that he had a liver that was easily palpable in his abdomen—hard, nodular, and non-tender. I do not remember any other physical characteristic. Nor do I remember his name or any aspect of his history. He was basically the first liver I palpated. At no point did I see him as a suffering patient needing any sort of recognition.

The mantra was "see one, do one, and then teach one." That was how I learned to do stitches in the ER. First you were an observer, then you spent some time practicing on an inanimate object, then you worked on a live human being. My very first time, I had to stitch lacerations on the face of a completely inebriated patient who required no anesthetic. It was an event filled with anxiety, but at least I did not have to worry about pain or discomfort.

At the time, there were no blood-drawing teams, and students helped the interns acquire the blood samples. I got so proficient that a drug addict would allow only me to draw blood from his one accessible vein. Steadily, I gained plenty of skills. At that time, students had more firsthand learning opportunities because there were fewer legal entanglements and fewer specialized services. I benefited from a lot of direct, if superficial, interactions with patients and became very comfortable examining patients' bodies, feeling no compunction about invading their intimate space.

During the internal medicine internship and residency, the operative words were work, work, work, and experience, experience, experience. The justification was that house staff needed a tremendous amount of time with patients in order to function independently in private practice. While this allowed students to refine their skills and gain confidence in patient care, the hours were inhumane and erratic, sometimes 36 hours at a time, totaling almost 120 hours per week. It was brutal. It left little time for reading journals, and in the end, the patient suffered.

In my three years in residency, there were two strikes by the house staff union, the Committee of Interns and Residents, demanding a cap of 90 hours per week. We were quickly stifled in our attempt to establish merely arduous—as opposed to inhumane—conditions. I was the representative for my hospital and was threatened by attendings who said I would never be able to practice medicine in New York if we continued to strike. It was a stressful situation for them since they had to take on more of the daily responsibilities while we were not available. We ourselves were anxious to get back to work to prevent a major deterioration in medical care, and a prolonged walkout was unthinkable. Still, we did what we could and received some support. At one point, when we were picketing outside a small, private hospital associated with my program, a truck pulled up with a supply of rats to be used for lab experimentation. The truckers would not cross our protest line and left the crates of animals on the street, showing their support for our demands. In the end, however, the hospitals had the clout and power to prevail. We caved in quite quickly, even my house staff, which was one of the last to return.

It would take more than a decade to obtain saner hours. Unfortunately, changes are often the outcome of catastrophes, rather than reason or compassion. What moved the system to change was the tragic story of Libby Zion, an eighteen-year-old college freshman who was being treated for stress with antidepressants. She went to New York Hospital, a well-respected, academic medical center, with flu symptoms. She was admitted with some "strange jerking motions" and was treated with an opioid. The combination of her antidepressant and the opioid was contraindicated but probably not well recognized at the time. Libby developed a potentially fatal case of serotonin syndrome with tremors and exceedingly high temperatures. Because of continued agitation, now related to the treatment regimen, she was restrained and given Haldol, which only made the situation worse. She had a cardiac arrest and died.

The residents taking care of her had been working for over twenty-four hours and had been kept very busy. Who is to blame for this tragic outcome? The physicians or the system? Medical errors by doctors-in-training, overworked and sleep-deprived, were frequent but not publicized. Ultimately, the physicians were given reprimands and allowed to keep their medical licenses. The episode made headlines because Libby's father was a lawyer who wrote for the *New York Times*. Libby died in 1984, but not until 1989 did New York pass a law restricting doctors-in-training to an eighty-hour workweek.

The house staff was overworked, but during my internship, I was put in even more dire straits. There was an intern missing in my group and my caseload doubled, causing my census of patients to become unmanageable. Thinking back, I realize I was only able to survive because of teamwork, not with my fellow trainees and our superiors, but with medical students and nurses sympathetic to my plight. As it became increasingly difficult to keep up with my daily workload, my chief resident chastised me for falling behind and was even talking about having me fired. I had two medical students working alongside me, and one became so outraged by the way I was treated that she went to the attending doctor to defend me against unjust charges. I have always been grateful to this student for her support. Then, there were the nurses who had been working on the wards for many years and knew so much more than I did about the care of patients. They were important teachers for me, and I held them in high esteem. I never put myself in a superior position. The old-school notion of the physician as an authoritarian figure never worked for me.

Needless to say, I did not have much time to develop relationships with my patients or empathy for their plight. Some patients were memorable only because they were readmitted to the hospital so frequently—not the most positive circumstances for developing a rapport. There was a teenage diabetic who was admitted to the hospital in diabetic ketoacidosis (DKA) on a regular basis. I became quite comfortable taking care of this life-threatening complication since I saw the patient at least three times in three months. What was odd to me was that he responded so quickly to treatment; it seemed that he improved even before I'd instituted insulin therapy. All he appeared to need was some fluids and calories, and he'd be gone from the hospital within two days. With this observation in mind, the third time he was admitted to me, I did not give him extra insulin, just IV fluids, including dextrose. He did fine with his usual insulin dosing and was ready for discharge in the customary two-day period. I expressed to the nurses my surprise at how easy it was to stabilize him. They let me know that he was a narcotic mule, bringing heroin into the hospital to sell to patients. He was so adept at insulin management that he could withhold his insulin and start going into DKA and then take insulin and fluids shortly before being admitted since he did not trust the ER to start DKA management quickly enough. I confronted him with these allegations, and after that, I never saw him again. Perhaps he miscalculated when he tried it again. Or he simply moved his business to another hospital.

It is revealing that my single opportunity for cultivating a relationship with a patient was given to me by a drug dealer. I was extremely busy, doing my job conscientiously, but with little connection to the human beings receiving my treatment. The ICU environment required me to distance myself from the patient and instead put all my focus on skillfully keeping the patient alive for the duration of my shift. No matter how sick the patient was or how hopeless the situation, I desperately worked to maintain life. If someone died, it was a failure, even when the outcome was inevitable. The idea of death was anathema.

Sometimes the never-say-die approach would work. When I was a resident at a private hospital, an eighty-year-old woman with diabetes was admitted for malignant lactic acidosis (a dangerous accumulation of lactic acid in the blood), caused by the anti-diabetic drug Phenformin (which was eventually taken off the market). After an intense eight hours of frequent lab testing and titrating bicarbonate drip, along with other unusual treatment modalities to terminate a runaway deadly process, the patient survived. Sometimes what looks like undue perseverance will pay off.

Emergency situations when a code was called were a time for house staff to learn about death and its inevitability. In the majority of those I experienced, the patient did not survive. I would leave an unsuccessful code and feel everything was done that could have been done. I was in training before Do Not Resuscitate (DNR) regulations were instituted, and we often found ourselves in hopeless situations. The medical consensus might be that calling the code and initiating emergency procedures was useless, but often the patient's family refused to accept the inevitable and demanded treatment.

On one occasion, I was doing rounds on the ward while a large family surrounded their very sick mother. I told them that their mother was not going to survive much longer, and the goal should be to keep her comfortable and peaceful. The family, however, could not accept this scenario. When she suddenly stopped breathing, they were overwhelmed and screamed that I had to save their mother. I ushered them out of the room and called a code simply so the family could feel that we had tried everything. With the code team there, I instituted a short, life-saving procedure for the benefit of the family rather than the patient. When I came out of the room and told them that we had not been able to save her, they were devastated, holding onto each other for comfort. It felt unnatural to try to resuscitate a patient when there was no chance of success. Luckily, futile codes have become less frequent with the institution of DNR orders, but at the time, the patient's quality of life or their mode of dying was of little concern.

All in all, my training gave me little time to develop connections with my patients. It was only when I began my fellowship that I really started to cultivate this aspect of my calling. There was more continuity of care, and my interactions became more meaningful. Suddenly, there was time to think and time to learn, time for myself without the enervating night calls. I had left my East Coast roots and moved boldly to Seattle and the University of Washington system. My interest in research had never become a passion, and I wanted to have as broad a clinical experience as possible within an academic setting.

An endocrinology fellowship can easily lead to an academic career with little attention to clinical skills. I was more than lucky to be based at the U.S. Public Health Service, which had a general endocrinology clinic servicing the people of a three-state area, including maritime workers and Native Americans. It was a treasure trove of unusual patients. I learned first-hand the importance of treating each patient as unique rather than part of a generic population.

For example, during my fellowship, there was a male in his twenties who had been seen at the clinic for years for significantly low potassium levels, which, if left untreated, could be fatal. In endocrinology, there are a host of adrenal hormone excess conditions that lead to hypokalemia. His workup did not reveal a primary adrenal problem, nor did he experience hypertension or changes in his body habitus (his weight and physique) due to adrenal excess syndromes. So he was being kept on a massive amount of potassium supplementation. I deduced that he must be losing potassium through his kidneys instead of resorbing potassium properly from the urine. My working diagnosis was Bartter's syndrome, even though this could not be proven by testing since the genetic tests that can pinpoint this transport problem were not available at the time. Accordingly, I prescribed a potassium-sparing diuretic that significantly reduced his need for potassium supplementation. Both the diagnosis and treatment lie entirely outside the field of endocrinology, and typically, endocrinologists will not consider it. They keep their focus on hormonal causes, and if these are not found, then the process of looking for solutions can come to a standstill. I feel fortunate that early in my career, I was given such unusual cases, for they helped prevent me from falling into this rut.

It was also my privilege to learn from a wonderful physician, Dr. Leonard, whose stolid linear analysis was always accompanied by pearls of wisdom. He was able to illuminate the broader context for his clinical decisions and offered me heuristic devices to aid me in diagnosis. One memorable case was a Native American woman who came into the hospital stuporous, with a high level of calcium. It is unusual for hyperparathyroidism to cause significant increases in calcium in the blood. Elevated levels due to cancer are more likely, requiring a major workup, and the results can take days to come back. But Dr. Leonard did not embark on this route. He looked at the patient and her lab work and, after speaking to her family, was able to deduce that she had milk alkali syndrome from having combined thiazide diuretics, which cause calcium retention, with an excessive ingestion of calcium in the form of Tums. The clue for the initial diagnosis was that her bicarbonate blood test was high, and afterwards, the family confirmed that she took massive amounts of Tums for indigestion. With this diagnosis, the treatment became hydration with normal saline IVs. A simple solution to an unusual situation. I have not seen a case of milk alkali since.

Clinical diagnosis became exciting, a challenging, sometimes surprising process of balancing possibilities, probabilities, and practicalities. There were enough rare diagnoses to stimulate me to consider the unusual, but plenty of the basic fare to ground me in the customary.

The diabetic clinic was well-run and gave me a real opportunity to develop long-term relationships with patients. The tools to manage diabetes were crude at the time and consisted of urine sugar monitoring by the patient and twenty-four-hour urine sugar collections sent to the lab to monitor long-term sugar control. In retrospect, these measurements were very poor indicators of how the patient was doing, so the best advice we were giving diabetic patients was regarding diet and exercise. I also quickly realized that I could help with their blood sugar control simply by listening to them describe their lives and the obstacles they faced. When the patients sensed I was truly interested, they felt more motivated to pursue good self-care. Some of them followed me into private practice to maintain this beneficial relationship. For one of them, this was a logistical nightmare since she was blind and had to travel twenty miles via public transportation to see me. Her needs might have been better met by a larger organization with more resources, but she only trusted me. There was another diabetic patient who was an elderly Aleut woman living on an island off the Alaska coast. She, too, wanted to keep seeing me, but this was a practical impossibility no matter how much she appreciated my care.

Other clinical experiences were also memorable and of great benefit. I spent a year at a pediatric endocrinology clinic at Seattle Children's Hospital, learning about growth disorders, as well as three months in an OBGYN clinic for infertility. I enjoyed gaining literacy in the diverse realms of endocrinological practice. At a thyroid clinic, I was able to fulfil a goal that was of particular importance to me—expanding the diagnostic tools available to endocrinologists. The difficulty of determining whether a thyroid nodule was benign or malignant had been unsettling to me. Imaging with radioactive iodine was very imprecise. When the lump did not take up iodine, the possibility of cancer increased, but most nodules would still be benign. During my residency, I met a thyroidologist who did open biopsies: the neck was locally anesthetized and, under sterile conditions, an incision was made to expose the thyroid mass and remove tissue. It was an invasive and time-consuming procedure and not generally accepted. I decided to initiate a fine needle aspirate program. The fine needle was more like drawing blood and did not require a lot of prep time; one just needed good palpation skills to feel the lump and get an adequate sample. There was also a learning curve for the pathologist reading a sample of thyroid cells since many thyroid cancers do not contain very aberrant cells. Some thyroid cancers are even hard to diagnose after the whole thyroid is removed.

The head of the thyroid clinic was a great doctor and teacher and was supportive of my thyroid nodule aspirate protocol. My very first thyroid aspirate was performed on an easily palpable nodule. I had read as much as I could to determine which needles to use and how to prepare the slides. The pathologist was onboard, willing to use samples of just thyroid cells to look for malignancy. The results of my first aspirate were positive for papillary thyroid cancer, which can be quite distinctive in the evaluation of the smears. Upon operation, the diagnosis of papillary thyroid cancer was confirmed. Everyone was impressed, and clinical attendings wanted to learn the thyroid aspirate protocol so they could start performing it too.

I was developing a lot of confidence with the procedure when, about a year later, my initial patient was in the clinic for a routine follow-up. His neck had some residual induration from the surgery, but I thought I felt a slight lump in the thyroid bed. I aspirated the area, and lo and behold, there were papillary thyroid cancer cells present. We re-operated on the patient, and a small amount of thyroid tissue was removed. A miniscule, maybe irrelevant amount of papillary cancer was found. I must admit that these early successes were a bit lucky, for in the years after, I have had many cases with ambiguous or even inadequate results. That is medicine—not an exact science!

CLINICAL PRACTICE, HERE I COME!

My private practice started humbly. My room, inside the office of another endocrinologist, was a converted storage closet, and together we made use of two exam rooms and a single employee. Within a year, we moved to better quarters, and thereafter, our physical space and medical team continued to grow. At the beginning, I would see not just endocrinologic patients but also general internal medicine referrals.

I found out that it took time to translate my extensive academic knowledge base into good clinical practice. I'm reminded of the Greek concept of phronesis, which refers to the wisdom that comes from experience, an accumulation of useful habits combined with ethical principles and good judgment. Aristotle made a point of distinguishing this quality from other intellectual virtues, and I find the distinction extremely useful.

Within the first month of practice, a woman in her twenties was referred to me for fatigue. This was not an uncommon occurrence since hormonal imbalances can often manifest as a lack of energy. After a complete history and physical, I felt an endocrinological problem was unlikely. Routine tests revealed a possible urinary tract infection, which I treated with an antibiotic. The patient came back a week later feeling worse. Now, I felt obliged to do some endocrinologic testing. Her thyroid was normal, and an adrenal stimulation test also came back normal. I was at a loss. Eventually, pregnancy became the obvious reason for the change in her well-being. She had a history of irregular periods, and presumably the referring doctor had ruled out pregnancy, so I did not initially pursue this course. The diagnosis was good news for the patient, and no harm had been done, except for some unnecessary tests and procedures.

Unfortunately, another patient did not have such a benign outcome. A woman in her late twenties came to me suffering from acute panic attacks as well as general anxiety. The primary care physician had referred her for possible pheochromocytoma (an adrenal tumor producing excessive hormones and neurotransmitters). My judgment was that pheochromocytoma testing was not needed and that her panic attacks could be treated with medication. She was not amenable to seeing a psychiatrist, and I decided that medication would be sufficient to treat her emotional distress. A couple of weeks later, she came into the office with a new complaint—piercing headaches. I did an eye exam and saw evidence of papilledema (swelling of the optic disc), suggesting increased pressure in the brain. I immediately admitted her to the hospital and called in a neurologist. A CAT scan was done showing a frontal lobe tumor, positioned in such a way that it might elude a routine exam. The tumor herniated, and the patient was dead within twenty-four hours of admission. The autopsy revealed that she had a high-grade glioblastoma that would not have been amenable to any treatment, but that was not much solace to me. It is not that every patient with a panic disorder needs a CAT scan to rule out a brain tumor, but rather that I needed to be more aware of that possibility when I developed my diagnostic plan. I was not sued, but I felt full of guilt and remorse for not having figured out her diagnosis earlier, regardless of the outcome.

While these mistakes are indelibly printed in my mind, the early years of my practice were largely filled with positive experiences as I cultivated strong relationships with my patients and refined my clinical acumen and skills. While diabetes was the major focus of my practice, thyroid nodule evaluation was a special area of interest. The investigations that began during my residency continued after I started my practice.

Early on, I visited the Karolinska Institute in Sweden, which boasted the world's largest series of thyroid aspirate results. I observed a clinic set up like an assembly line, with aspirations performed one after the other. Sometimes, the nodules were not even palpable, but still the procedure was performed because the patient had been referred for it. The doctor doing the procedure had no experience with the patient and could refer only to the history provided on the consult form. Nor would the doctor follow up with the patient once the results were back. I knew right away that this was not the way I wanted to practice.

However, I did obtain a good thyroid aspirating gun to perform procedures more easily, as well as a detailed, illustrated manual of thyroid aspirate cellular pathologies, which I gave to my hospital's pathologist. Obtaining the aspirate was usually the easy part. The interpretation of the individual cells and their patterns could be difficult. Probably, as much as a quarter of the results were indeterminate. Then I was back to relying on clinical experience to determine what to say and do.

A thyroid nodule emergency is unusual, even if cancer is involved. But a doctor must always be open to the unexpected. This is one of the lessons of practical experience. In one case, a woman in her thirties was referred for a thyroid mass that was very evident visually. The lump was relatively soft, which suggested a cystic fluid mass rather than a firmer thyroid tissue mass. The thyroid aspiration did not elicit any fluid, a surprising result, so I was eager to see the report.

Two days later, the findings showed sheets of lymphocytes mixed with thyroid cells. The common diagnosis would have been Hashimoto's thyroiditis, but the soft texture of the mass and the preponderance of lymphocytes present alerted me to the worrisome possibility of a lymphoma. The patient was called by my medical assistant,

Patty, who noticed that the patient was talking very hoarsely. Without hanging up the phone, Patty interrupted my meeting with another patient to sound the alarm. I instructed her to call an ambulance to bring the patient immediately to the ER.

Lymphomas of the thyroid can grow very rapidly and basically strangle the patient. I called the ER to let the physician know that a patient would be arriving soon, needing a tracheotomy with an open biopsy of the mass to alleviate suffocation. An emergency thyroidectomy was not needed, however, since radiation therapy would succeed in shrinking the lymphoma quickly. This was my only case of a primary lymphoma of the thyroid, and I developed a lot of respect for its dangerous swiftness. Fortunately, all other times that I palpated a soft thyroid mass, fluid was present. Lightning does not strike twice.

Ultimately, I expanded my ability to aspirate barely palpable nodules by being certified in thyroid ultrasound. This technology proved very useful. A friend of mine developed a big neck mass, and I initially aspirated over 20cc of a clear fluid, but this was before the days of ultrasound, and the mass recurred and was even bigger. Using ultrasound, I was able to completely drain it, removing 300cc of fluid, and it never returned.

While this new technology would appear to be invaluable for precise sampling and diagnosis, it has also led to many dilemmas. There are simply too many thyroid lumps found by ultrasound for it to be practical to biopsy them all. The probability of finding cancer is small. Many patients were referred to me when CTs and MRIs, done for other reasons, revealed thyroid masses. It was often hard to reason with these patients about the inutility of doing an aspirate. Using ultrasound, I could now aspirate nodules in a way that was impossible before, but the truth is, these hard-to-feel nodules are rarely malignant. A wait-and-see attitude is advisable, but this can be hard for patients to accept. Technological advance has made so many tools available to us. Still, we must still exercise judgment in their use. If we did CTs and MRIs on everyone, and then performed aspirates for all the nodules discovered, the situation would get untenable, even absurd.

These are just a few examples of the learning that comes with experience. Certainly, a doctor's education never stops. Over my career,

I attended sixty to seventy clinical investigator meetings and annual American Diabetes Association meetings and kept abreast of ongoing developments in my field and elsewhere via the medical literature. Even as I worked in a clinical setting, I continued to conduct research to learn about the conditions I was treating. For example, it was general wisdom that a clear fluid aspirate would suggest a parathyroid cyst, not of thyroid origin. I set up a protocol so that whenever I had a pure clear fluid aspirate, the specialty lab would run a parathormone assay that was developed for non-blood assays. Four out of five aspirates did indeed have sky-high parathormone levels. I was able to confirm my clinical diagnosis with lab findings.

By the time I retired, the field of aspirates had evolved even further, with the use of genetic markers to help diagnose malignancy. A practicing doctor must adapt to a continually evolving field, exercising judgment and refining their clinical experience. Diagnosis, too, is a skill that a doctor must continue to hone, and as I have mentioned, mistakes are made along the way.

MALPRACTICE

Medical decision-making is permeated by uncertainty. On the other hand, physicians should be held accountable for mistakes that are flagrant. Litigation plays an important role in this regard.

I find it interesting that missed diagnoses lead to more legal suits than procedural errors. My malpractice coverage costs as an endocrinologist were as high as those of cardiologists, whose procedures are much more invasive. Of course, the legal system helps rectify as well as deter egregious errors, but in the United States, which has by far the highest number of malpractice claims in the world, the balance has tipped too far in the direction of tenuous claims.

No physician wants to be sued for missing a diagnosis, so they often order tests even when they are fairly certain that the results will be negative. Clinical judgment often takes a backseat to the fear of legal repercussions. The easy road is to test excessively rather than employ the clinical acumen that physicians have gained over time. Needless to say, I, along with some of my colleagues, prefer the latter course.

I was personally never sued for an error, but since the threat of suits has such an impact on the day-to-day decision-making of medical practice today, I'd like to share some of my stories from the realm of jurisprudence.

I'll start with an example of a dubious suit. For several years, I was in a call group with an endocrinologist, an internist, and two gastro-enterologists. One weekend while on call, I was following a patient seen by one of my partners for anticoagulation management because he had developed deep vein thrombosis, or clotting, after knee surgery. The patient was otherwise young and healthy. My task was to monitor the anticoagulation parameters to determine the amount of blood thinner to be administered—enough for a therapeutic response but not so much as to cause excess bleeding. When I examined the patient's calf that had the clot, I noted that while the calf looked all right, there was increased swelling, heat, and tenderness in the oper-ated knee joint. I was concerned about an infection in the joint as a potential postop complication. This was an urgent problem, and I wanted the knee aspirated before I started IV antibiotics. The ortho-pedist on call did the procedure, and antibiotics were initiated. There was indeed a staph infection, and the patient recovered after getting antibiotics and went home.

The patient, however, was irate and sued the orthopedist who per-formed the procedure, in addition to the covering orthopedist who had seen the patient earlier in the day without noting the possibility of infection, and the internist for whom I was covering. Interestingly, I was not sued because I had sounded the alarms. The legal case was all about how much permanent disability the patient had suffered because of a possible delay in the treatment of the staph infection. My suspicion was that he was more emotionally affected than physically. It's hard to say when, in the days following his procedure, the clinical suspicion of an infection could have been raised.

Then there are the legitimate lawsuits due to error. The most egre-gious case I witnessed regarded a young man admitted with advanced diabetic ketoacidosis while I was on ER backup. He had no previous history of diabetes but had been seen at a quick medical clinic for fatigue, weight loss, and a possible upper respiratory infection. The examination at that time was cursory, without lab work or consideration given to his weight loss, increased urination, and profound weakness. He was given an antibiotic, which did not help, so he returned to the clinic five days later. At that point, because of increased urination, a urine test was done that showed glucose in the urine. Blood was drawn, and he was discharged from the clinic, awaiting results. The next day, the results showed florid diabetic ketoacidosis (DKA), a dangerous build-up of acids in the blood, and he was told to go to the hospital immediately.

I was initially confident that he would do fine with intensive treatment. I knew that DKA could be life-threatening, but I had always been able to right the ship in the past. I spent sixteen hours straight with him, and still, he did not stabilize. No matter which maneuvers I performed, nothing could resolve the malignant acidotic state, which then combined with lactic acidosis to become utterly unmanageable. The young wife was there throughout the night, and I kept in continual communication with her during this vigil. I tried to explain to her the problems we were having stabilizing her husband, giving her context by describing the physiologic dysfunction that was occurring. Never before had I felt so hopeless and frustrated taking care of a patient. It broke my heart to see this twenty-year-old woman, who had a young child, suddenly lose her husband when it would not have happened if the physician at the clinic had paid attention to the whole patient during his first visit.

In the subsequent lawsuit, which was easily won, I acted as witness since I was one of the physicians involved in his care as well as an expert in diabetes. I had only known his wife for that one night, but we had developed a bond. She thanked me for the care and dedication I had exhibited while taking care of her husband. I felt buoyed by her faith in me but dejected by my inability to save her husband's life. Could I have done something better? As a physician, one can't help but ask oneself such questions.

Other legitimate lawsuits, while not as heartbreaking, still provoke outrage. I'm speaking of the unscrupulous physicians who are out to make a profit while hoodwinking the populace. I was involved in one such case when the State of Washington decided to investigate the practices of an obesity mill. It was the era of phentermine-fenfluramine, or phen-fen, a combination of medications that could achieve some weight loss but eventually was determined to cause cardiac valvular deformities.

Before this toxicity was well-publicized, the combination was prescribed to patients without official FDA approval. All weight-loss medications have side effects and should be used only in the case of morbid obesity, when the benefits may outweigh the risks, but still, patients who are just slightly overweight will clamor for the drugs. I occasionally prescribed the phen-fen combination, using the strict criteria of morbid obesity combined with the comorbidity of diabetes. As soon as the study was published revealing the valvular heart disease, I called the few patients who were taking the medication and had them stop immediately.

The doctor with the "obesity mill" was prescribing the medication to anyone who would pay for it. There were hundreds of patients, some of whom even had ideal body weight. He performed extensive blood screening using his own lab, without addressing most of the abnormalities found and sometimes commenting incorrectly on the results. He was also selling phen-fen directly out of his office. He had his patients come in for frequent monitoring, which was completely meaningless but of course very lucrative. At no point did he inform them of the risks they were taking. I was outraged and ready to testify in court about this scam, but lawyers were able to get him off without a trial, and all he lost was his Washington State license.

The whole episode left a bad taste in my mouth. Here was a physician representing the worst in medical care, and in the end, he received a slap on the wrist. I can't help but question the current state of our legal system. It instills so much fear that good, competent physicians feel compelled to perform countless, unnecessary tests. Then, when an avaricious physician performs a heinous act—a glaring example of malpractice, legally and morally—the verdict is utterly inadequate.

This is a clear example of how doctors can go astray. The need to exercise good judgment is, of course, a broader issue, and I would like now to return to trends that are even more significant in affecting the course of medicine today. A historical overview showed us that science has not always dominated the field. The idea that science delivers the truth is exciting and empowering; at one point, it was revolutionary. But it can also foster complacency and distract doctors from the continual need to exercise their good judgment as well as delve into realms beyond the purview of science.

THE SCIENCE

"The saddest aspect of life now is that science gathers knowledge faster than society gathers wisdom."

Isaac Asimov

CHAPTER THREE

Science, Its Value and Limitations

Science, from the Latin word *scientia,* or knowledge, is the systematic study of the natural world via observation and experiment. Prior to the scientific revolution, information was accepted on faith, and the field of medicine was plagued with erroneous theories and practices. Since then, scientific development has improved healthcare in ways we cannot begin to count. But does this mean that the practice of medicine is above all a science? Certainly, this idea dominated my training as a medical student. And I continue to have a deep reverence for science and deplore the ways in which our culture, despite the rise of science, remains unscientific and irrational.

We have no problem clinging to beliefs that contradict the evidence. Alex Berezow, a microbiologist and editor of *RealClearScience,* explores this phenomenon, which crosses partisan lines. While Republicans are accused of being unscientific because of the attacks on evolutionary theory by a vocal minority, Democrats are more likely to be against GMOs, despite assurances regarding their safety by the National Academy of Sciences. Then, there is the antivax movement, which puts the entire population at risk. In contrast, one of the most spiritual among us, the Dalai Lama, has a keen interest in scientific investigations and has stated if science can prove one of his Buddhist precepts to be incorrect, he will bow to the evidence.

I do not hold with the distortions of truth that come from a misunderstanding of science and its methods. At the same time, I don't believe in automatically accepting everything propounded in the name of science. All advancement of knowledge is based on data leading to high quality evidence, but the collection of information is not accomplished in a vacuum and reflects the predispositions and values of the investigators. While the ideal is objectivity, bias is inevitable. And this is where wisdom must enter. Only when we are willing to admit the limitations, of ourselves and our knowledge, can science play its appropriate role.

My purpose in this part of the book is to explore the limitations of science in the medical field. To do so, we must look more closely at what we mean by science and scientific rigor. According to the philosopher Michael Strevens, science advances only by application of the "iron rule," which he defines as follows:

1. Strive to settle all arguments by empirical testing.
2. To conduct an empirical test to decide between a pair of hypotheses, perform an experiment or measurement, one of whose possible outcomes can be explained by one hypothesis (and accompanying cohort) but not the other. (Strevens, 2020, p.96)

A key tenet of the scientific enterprise is falsifiability, which originated in the 1930s with the theorist Karl Popper. The idea is that for a theory to be scientific, it must be falsifiable. If a theory cannot be turned into a falsifiable statement, it can never be tested empirically. Thus, a statement like "Hydroxycholoroquine is a treatment for COVID-19" can be falsified by a series of studies testing its efficacy. On the other hand, a statement such as "God exists" is not falsifiable. The work of scientists is confined to falsifying theories. This requirement narrows the scope of investigation considerably, as we shall see later. Also, no investigation can ever be definitive. The more studies there are that do not prove your idea false, the more likely it is to be true; nonetheless, this truth remains provisional.

In fact, science, if it is rigorous, is constantly revising its formulations. We can never accept anything as definitively true because in the future, new data may revise it. The philosopher Thomas Kuhn coined the famous phrase "paradigm shift" to highlight the malleability of science. Studies are performed that conform to the current dogma, but eventually, something is proven false, and the underlying tenets must be reworked. There's a shift to a new paradigm, which holds true till new evidence contradicts it.

The iconic paradigm shift of the twentieth century was the passing of the torch from Newton to Einstein. Newtonian laws regarding mass, forces, and motion were replaced by Einstein's theory of relativity, and absolutes (other than the speed of light) were discarded in favor of conditional relationships between space and time. The vocabulary of certainty was replaced by relativity. Observations needed to be qualified, and the world became a lot more mysterious.

Then, quantum mechanics appeared on the scene, with mathematics becoming the primary means of describing the world. Scientific doctrines had to be reevaluated yet again, and the revelations were not always well received. Einstein was disturbed by the phenomenon of quantum entanglement, when an action performed on one of two spatially distant particles affects the other. He labelled it "spookiness at a distance."

Once a new paradigm is established, other avenues are ignored or even ridiculed. This is, of course, highly unscientific. A true scientist understands the inherent limits of science, understands that something is only ever tentatively true, and that data must continue to be gathered. In fact, the scientific method requires the accumulation of voluminous amounts of data, for only in this way is the likelihood of a statement being true increased, very gradually and over time.

To me, the ultimate question is what kind of universe are we inhabiting? Is it one that we can know in an absolute way? Or is it one that remains in essence mysterious because there is always the potential to discover more? This dichotomy is encapsulated for me by the contrasting views of two famous scientists: Sean Carroll and David Bohm. Carroll claimed that "the laws of physics underlying everyday life are completely known" (Carroll, 2017, p.177). In contrast, his fellow physicist Bohm posited that "whatever we say anything is, it isn't" (Bohm, 1987, p.133). I know this sounds like a perverse statement that gets us nowhere, but it basically tells us that we will inevitably be proven wrong, and that is, logically and scientifically, true.

And it is also profoundly liberating and inspiring. In the words of Thoreau, "the universe is wider than our views of it" (Thoreau, 2004, p.309). If we truly believe this, pursuing alternatives becomes easier and exciting. Einstein once told a friend of his who was a physician that "the gift of fantasy has meant more to me than my talent for absorbing positive knowledge" (Janos, 1947, p.207). In the field of medicine, cultivating an open mind is critical. There is no dearth of data. The randomized clinical trial rules the day, and there are tests for every condition. But all of this information must be navigated, and the doctor caring for the individual patient is given no clear and definitive answers. Science, while it floods us with evidence, cannot tell us what to do.

RANDOMIZED CLINICAL TRIALS: RIGOR AND RIGIDITY

The buzzword these days is evidence-based medicine, and the best evidence-based medicine is produced by the randomized clinical trial, or RCT. What makes these studies so important and compelling is the attempt to eliminate human fallibility, the subjectivity of both investigator and patient.

RCTs follow an exceedingly rigid design protocol. First, there must be a precise formulation of the treatment and its objectives regarding causality. It is crucial that the endpoint be defined before the study is launched, not after, because the study's design depends on it. The data produced cannot be used later to prove other phenomena. The study is set up to compare two groups that are recruited equally but treated differently: the active intervention group and the control group, usually given a placebo or an already approved medication for comparison. The inclusion and exclusion criteria for participants must be carefully defined. The goal is to get rid of factors that could skew the outcome. Both groups must be balanced as to demographics (age, sex, ethnic background), disease state, comorbidities, and co-medications. Patients cannot know which group they belong to, and the investigators must be blind to this as well. Sample size is predetermined to maximize the study's chance of a successful outcome—too few patients and the effect will not be proven, especially if it's small. This protocol has been systematized by the CONSORT Group (Consolidated Standards of Reporting Trials), which has created an itemized checklist of the criteria that must be met.

Clearly, designing and implementing RCTs correctly can be a Herculean task. I personally have been involved in hundreds of studies. After practicing endocrinology for ten years, I decided to venture into clinical research as a way of engaging in cutting-edge work, investigating various medical disorders, especially diabetes in all its facets—testing, insulins, new hypoglycemic agents, and technological devices, from continuous glucose monitors to closed loop insulin systems. With two other endocrinologists, I founded the Rainier Clinical Research Center (RCRC), which participated in hundreds of randomized clinical trials under the auspices of several large pharmaceutical companies. Over a twenty-five-year period, I developed a deep awareness of the intricacies of validating the efficacy and safety of medications and procedures as well as great respect and gratitude for the continual accrual of scientific data. Obviously, doctors want to help their patients by using all the information available.

And the amount of information is phenomenal. According to data in Pub Med Trend, in the last fifty years, over a half million RCTs were documented. But the quality and significance of this work varies widely. John Ioannidis, in a landmark study in 2005, investigated how frequently studies were contradicted or modified over time. He reviewed a group of respected, highly cited studies between 1990 and 2003, one hundred and fifteen in total, and found that only forty-nine met the standards necessary for his analysis. Of these, four studies showed negative results while seven studies were subsequently contradicted. Seven showed lessened effects in repeat studies, twenty were replicated, and eleven had gone unchallenged. Thus, of the crème de la crème studies, only a bit more than half stood the test of time.

According to a comprehensive review by Dr. Prasad et al. of the research studies submitted to the *New England Journal of Medicine* from 2001 to 2010, 40% suggested abandoning present-day, standard medical practices for previous treatments and only 38% reaffirmed established practices. Certainly, given that the results of any RCT may be overturned by a subsequent trial, the importance of replication is clear. But even when this is done, the picture only becomes more complicated. A new study with a new design and execution as well as different results is simply adding more information without necessarily changing the validity of the previous study. Which one is right? Do three studies break the tie?

As a practicing physician, I often found myself pontificating on the importance of controlling cholesterol, investigating with my patients the various treatment options, detailing the evidence from various sources. The exercise would become vertiginous, and eventually, I would have to bring the patient and myself back to the ground, saying, "Don't get too caught up by my ranting and all these numbers since five years from now, my facts will change. What's important is that we still be here together, learning from each other about how to best take care of your health."

Given the divergence of results among RCTs, it seems that meta-analyses might play an important role in determining a course of action. Statistically, conclusions are stronger when there is more data, and a statistical analysis of a whole group of well-done RCTs can give greater weight to a certain conclusion. Unfortunately, it is often impossible to make statistically valid comparisons since the studies almost inevitably diverge in their criteria. And any analysis of these scientifically rigorous trials will be vulnerable to bias and interpretation. Even if we are full of integrity and strive to be neutral, we still have our ideas and preferences, and what we observe is not necessarily what's there. As Einstein remarked during a lecture by Heisenberg in 1926, "whether you can observe a thing or not depends on the theory which you use. It is the theory which decides what can be observed."

Another big issue is outcome-reporting bias, meaning that only positive or interesting results are published, not negative or mundane findings. If a study shows no beneficial effect, there is less incentive to publish it. It is hard to fault a journal for wanting to include only provocative and confirming evidence in their august pages. This bias is inevitable, and we need to be aware of how our overall picture is skewed as a result. Recently, standards have been put in place to correct for this bias, but that will improve our picture in the future; we continue to rely on studies from the past.

In truth, the design, implementation, interpretation, as well as dissemination of RCTs is riddled with challenges and pitfalls. I have not yet addressed the role of statistics. There is no data without statistics. Data is accumulated and analyzed statistically to give it heft and meaning. But statistics can mislead. Mark Twain liked to say, "There are three kinds of lies: Lies, Damned Lies, and Statistics" (Twain, 1907, p.471). An outcome might have statistical significance and still not be true. And conversely, something may have been shown to have no statistical significance and still be important.

I'm reminded of a conversation I had during a global medical exchange trip. When we stopped in the Soviet Union, we never did get to talk to any physicians. Instead, we were met by bureaucrats, all extolling the virtues of Soviet medical care. One of them boasted that in the USSR there were zero suicides. I could not help but ask how that was possible. The reply was that there were no statistics showing suicide. Clearly, statistical measures were prized to the point of absurdity, so revered as the ultimate lens on reality that what they did not reveal simply did not exist.

This story also introduces the question of bias. While statistics are supposed to yield a conclusion that is scientifically sound, there is, in the case of every study, the question of who is doing the study and what their motives are. A study may appear to be rigorous, but it is so easy for bias to sneak into its design. A survey of two thousand psychologists, asking them to rate their usage of questionable research practices, revealed that fully two thirds excluded measured outcome variables that might not support their desired conclusions. The fact that the investigators were willing to admit these shortcomings suggests that human subjectivity is accepted as an inevitable pitfall. Perhaps that is why we even have an acronym—QRP—for questionable research practices. Though they can never be condoned, they are here to stay. (John et al., 2012, p.524).

With every study that yields statistically significant results, we must entertain the possibility that the dice were loaded, the study designed so as to yield the positive value. Often, statistics are used to compare one company's drug with that of their competitor. Clearly, the goal driving these studies is not the patient's well-being since that would be served more or less by both drugs, but the companies' desire to increase their relative market share. This same drive is responsible for the excess of marketing we see. Both the studies and the marketing add tremendously to the cost of the drug. While one might be impressed by the wealth of data generated, it is not in service of the patient.

Even if there were no bias or distortion, the results give a skewed picture of the reality that doctors face. Life is not uniform; often, what appears extraordinary is really on the outer fringes of the ordinary. But in an RCT, individual results lose their significance. Experimenters are not interested in outliers or exceptions to the rule. They aggregate the data and homogenize participants to get rid of confounding variables. Individual results may be interesting and relevant to the individual patients, but the more their numbers veer, the more they interfere with the drive to reach conclusions of statistical significance. The RCT, in order to test a hypothesis about a group, deliberately minimizes the importance of results that diverge. It thereby offers a falsely uniform picture compared to the rich variety of patients that a practicing physician encounters.

What is statistically significant may not be clinically significant. The reality is that physicians must make a lot of decisions for which there is little or no statistically significant evidence. RCTs, by virtue of their very design, do not reflect society at large. Physiological response to a medication will depend on a multitude of factors, including ethnicity, gender, belief systems, and social status, and the conclusions of any study apply only to the population selected. Unfortunately, because the design of the trial needs to address adequate sample size, recruit subjects who meet all the eligibility criteria, and maintain appropriate quality control procedures, often, by the time the study has been made to conform to all the criteria, its results have become so narrowly defined that they are no longer useful for the population at large. The acronym WEIRD (Western, Educated, Industrialized, Rich, and Democratic), coined by Joseph Henrich, describes the populations of many of the most revered RCTs. Women have often been excluded, as have Black and Indigenous people. Age and health status continue to be severely restricted. Altogether, by focusing on the internal validity of the trial, scientists sacrifice applicability, or generalizability. Often, the intervention that was studied so rigorously never enters the real world of medical practice.

The trials do not provide an accurate picture of the reality of medical practice for another reason. The participants are treated differently than they would be in the real world. The volunteers are paid and monitored meticulously to assure that they take the medications exactly as prescribed and are questioned regularly as to adverse events. Also, the placebo effect is deliberately minimized, even though in a clinical setting a doctor might use it for added benefit.

I'd like to address the value of longitudinal studies in this context. Observational studies do not meet the criteria defining RCTs, and yet they have been a great boon to medicine by generating further research on a host of topics. Compared to RCTs, they require extended periods of time to yield meaningful conclusions. The Framingham Heart Study, focused on the epidemiology of arteriosclerotic heart disease, is an ongoing study that began in 1948. The format is a prospective cohort study, tracking multiple variables for a cohort from a small town in Massachusetts. The study led to the identification of multiple risk factors for cardiovascular disease, including cigarette smoking, uncontrolled hypertension, hyperlipidemia, and menopause. Such effects of longer duration elude RCTs, which are extremely expensive to maintain and usually have timelines of less than a year.

Another major example is the Nurses' Health Study involving over 120,000 married nurses between the ages of thirty and fifty-five. Established in 1976, it continued into the mid-1980s, and the collection of data was changed and refined as findings dictated. Initially, the focus was on contraceptive use, smoking, cancer, and cardiovascular disease. Diet and nutrition were added after the first couple of years. In 1989, the Nurses' Health Study 2 was initiated, including more detailed data on exercise and food intake. And in 2010, the Growing Up Today (GUTS) study followed 25,000 children of previously enrolled NHS 2 participants. A tremendous amount was learned regarding the increased risk of diabetes due to smoking, obesity, lack of exercise, and the consumption of trans fats. The risk of ovarian cancer decreased with the use of oral contraceptives, but that of breast cancer increased, depending on the contraceptive. There were many other findings, requiring further study for verification and elucidation. In the end, the amount of data obtained was extraordinary, and researchers have been kept busy for years, unpacking and validating the various findings in a more controlled fashion.

All observational studies include a diversity of participants while they set up some initial age criteria and some other defining factor, such as living in Framingham or being a nurse (usually white female). Thus, the conclusions will not apply to the whole population, and yet the studies tend to be more diverse than RCTs and generalizable. A tremendous amount of information is generated, sometimes over decades, that can reveal previously unknown avenues of inquiry.

A pioneer in the individual observation approach was Dr. Theodore Pincus, who amassed an impressive amount of clinical data on his rheumatologic patients using, in an era before computerization, consecutive patient self-report questionnaires. His rationale was that "any clinical encounter in which a single 'best' approach is not known—the situation of most encounters between health professionals and patients—may be viewed as a potential opportunity for scientific inquiry." In fact, such inquiry "should be viewed as a legitimate, and even necessary, scientific endeavor" (Pincus, 1997, p.19). Dr. Pincus meticulously inputted all this data over decades. The information was helpful for the doctor-patient visit itself as well as for integrated analysis later. The data of serial lab tests and medications was also included. Of course, there are problems with collecting data in this way, particularly with the reliability and recall of patients. Still, a true-to-life clinical experience is being utilized to further knowledge, not the restricted artificial setting of RCTs. And outliers can be noted and addressed.

We must be careful not to dismiss studies such as these simply because they do not adhere to the rigorous standards that govern RCTs. Their results do not lose all validity. I'm reminded of the first rudimentary trial for scurvy. It did not pass scientific muster by any means, and yet its conclusions were correct and heeding them saved lives. Sometimes, a too rigorous adherence to the criteria of RCTs can have tragic consequences, as was seen in the 1980s when extracorporeal membrane oxygenation (ECMO) was being explored as a novel way of treating respiratory failure in infants. The team that first studied it chose to apply the Zelen algorithm, developed by the biostatistician Marvin Zelen and based on gambling theory—the rule is to play the winner. The physicians were concerned about the ethics of "withholding an unproven but potentially lifesaving treatment," and the Zelen algorithm allowed them to assign subjects to the more successful treatment. The strategy resulted in one infant being assigned the "conventional" treatment and dying, and eleven infants in a row being assigned the experimental ECMO treatment, all of them surviving. After the end of the official study, ten additional infants met the criteria for ECMO treatment. Eight were treated with ECMO, and all eight survived. Two were treated conventionally, and both died. Still, there was controversy because the study had not been randomized in the conventional way. A proper RCT was performed that reconfirmed the efficacy of ECMO. But it was only stopped after another four babies died, having been denied the new treatment, while the rest survived. I am not advocating for the Zelen algorithm to be used widely. It will in many cases be inefficient or improperly utilized. Yet, when this method is applicable and beneficial, to reject it out of allegiance to a predetermined set of standards is tragic.

In a similar way, the FDA's rigor around drug approval at times can run counter to patients' interests. Often, new medications must pass through an inordinate number of studies before they are approved. Meanwhile the treatment is delayed (often when it is already available in Europe), and patients are deprived of much needed care. Then, there's the cost, which gets factored into the cost of the medication. Research and development is expensive!

TESTS: A MATTER OF INTERPRETATION

Not only has scientific endeavor provided us with a wealth of data to explain disease and its treatment, but it has also made possible the use of innumerable tests to help doctors diagnose their patients. But as in the case of RCTs, test results in and of themselves are not enough. They can be misleading, and patients can often misinterpret findings and draw erroneous conclusions.

First, it is important to remember that tests are not 100% accurate. Consider a test with a false-positive rate of 5%, meaning that 5% of tests lead to a false positive. In general, this is not a bad rate, but it is horrible for a disease with a low prevalence. For example, if prevalence is one in one thousand and the false-positive rate is 5%, then screening a thousand people will lead to fifty false positives and only one true positive. This means that if you take the test and are positive, there's only a 2% chance that you have the disease. Hardly good odds. Thus, blanket testing often makes no sense.

Most tests are described in terms of their sensitivity and specificity. Sensitivity is the ability of a test to correctly identify patients who have the disease. A 100% sensitive test has no false negatives (FN)—it will reveal all the people who have the disease, true positives (TP)—but it will also include false positives (FP). Such a test is good for screening, but if there are a lot of false positives, a lot of patients will be treated who don't have the condition. Specificity is the ability of a test to correctly identify those who do *not* have the disease. A 100% specific test has no false positives—it will reveal all the people who do not have the disease, true negatives (TN)—but it will also include false negatives, so there could be a significant number of diseased patients who don't get diagnosed. How reassuring is that?

Sensitivity= TP/(TP+FN)
Sensitivity is 100% if the number of false negatives is zero.

Specificity= TN/(TN+FP)
Specificity is 100% if there are no false positives.

The PSA test for prostate cancer can be a very sensitive test, picking up most prostate cancers but with a specificity low enough to include many false positives, leading to unnecessary and potentially harmful invasive procedures. The cutoff point for a prostate cancer workup can vary from 4 to 10. But the vast number of PSAs in that range represent prostate cancers that are slow-growing, and the patient is often likely to outlive the malignancy without treatment. Also, remember that many of these intermediate PSA values may be false positives. Thus, the patient who has been tested can find himself in a waiting game fraught with uncertainty. Say I have a PSA of 8. Should I wait and redraw a PSA in six months or one year? Should I get a prostatic biopsy with a slight potential of a post-procedure bleed or infection, when only about one out of three biopsies will be positive? To add to the complexity, there are other diagnostic aids such as a free PSA test or PSA velocity and doubling time. No wonder the official USPS Task Force does not recommend annual PSA testing!

How do all the numbers add up? It's easy to get lost, and statistics are often misinterpreted. For example, the efficacy of a vaccine, at say 95%, does not tell us the vaccinated individual's chance of getting COVID-19 since this depends on how much of the virus is around. If the prevalence rate is 10% of the population, then the risk of the vaccinated person is 95% lower, or 5% x 10%= .5%—extremely low. If there is a spike in COVID-19 cases to 20% of the population, the risk would double to a whopping 1%.

Statistics can tell us about the relative frequency of an event when a trial is repeated, but such information in isolation may be of little use. Bayesian statistics, a more nuanced approach, allows us to use other information to assess probability. It puts the information in a wider context. For example, the probability of a test being right is increased by identifying patients as high-risk, given the history of the patient and an examination. Doing tests in a void can be very unproductive and potentially misguided. If a coin tossed shows heads ten times in a row, should you still say the eleventh toss has a 50% chance of a head? Or should you consider the possibility that some other variable is involved? Tests by themselves are of limited value, whereas a doctor can bring to bear all kinds of extra information and understanding. For Dr. Siddhartha Mukherjee, the role of doctor is so important in this situation that it inspired one of his three laws of medicine: "A strong intuition is much more powerful than a weak test" (Mukherjee, 2015, p.22).

Even then, the process is fraught with uncertainty. I marshaled all that I knew in tackling a personal situation—reason, intuition, data, historical context—and I still don't know if I charted the right course. I have personally had the PSA test every year, contrary to the official recommendation, and perhaps that is where I went wrong. My annual PSAs for four years were steady. Then, six months after a probable prostatitis that I treated as a UTI, I had my PSA done, and it had risen over 50%. I had an ultrasound to rule out a bladder outlet obstruction, which would increase the risk of a UTI; it only showed a significant prostate enlargement. I was asymptomatic and decided to wait three months and repeat the PSA and get a free PSA test as well. Lo and behold, the PSA had increased another 30%, and the free PSA indicated moderate chance of cancer. Why was the PSA continuing to increase so dramatically? I was asymptomatic, with no evidence of an inflammatory cause. My thoughts kept going back to cancer. My urologist was on the fence and preferred that I get an MRI instead of a biopsy with its risk of a procedural morbidity. In the end, the MRI showed a large prostate and no cancer. Had I caused myself a lot of worry for nothing? I was making reasonable decisions each step of the way, but the whole process was fraught with uncertainty since the PSA does not give an answer, just information. Perhaps I should not have had the test in the first place, but once I knew the result, was I wrong to proceed? These are the questions for which there is no scientific answer. The dance with uncertainty is a very human one and beyond the ken of science.

The rate of breast cancer among women is similar to the rate of prostate cancer among men, affecting about one in eight women during their lifetime. The repercussions of untreated breast cancer, however, are more dire, and mammograms are extremely important. Even so, it makes sense to exercise judgment before proceeding with biopsies and surgery. The United States Preventive Services Task Force came out with the controversial recommendation that mammograms be biennial—performed every two years as opposed to annually—to decrease the percentage of false positives. Women with benign disease were able to avoid procedures with complications as well as the stress of worrying about cancer when none was present. Unfortunately, women who were not menopausal had more aggressive breast cancer, and waiting an extra year to be tested led to the discovery of larger tumors (although whether this was the cause of more death was undetermined). For post-menopausal women, the recommendation continues to make sense since there is some evidence that conducting biennial exams reduces radiation exposure. Nonetheless, cancer is such an emotionally charged issue that many women may still opt for annual screening, as well as biopsies and surgery, even when other data—the evaluation of risk factors, genetics, family history, etc.—do not suggest a heightened probability.

As my own experience demonstrated, tests and follow-up tests, just like the RCTs that generated them, may fail to give us the answers we crave. They are by no means as definitive as we'd like. They are what Dr. Faith Fitzgerald called a "punctilious quantification of the amorphous." Doctors who want to make use of them must do their best to exercise good judgment and combine what they learn with close observation of the individual patient. Even then, definitive answers will elude them.

CHAPTER FOUR

Navigating the Science in My Field

In the field of endocrinology, doctors address a range of concerns, most commonly, high cholesterol, hypertension, diabetes, estrogen, and osteoporosis. Each of these conditions is complex, and the science is continually evolving. Throughout my time as an endocrinologist, I always tried to be aware of the limitations of RCTs and of the guidelines that are derived from them, as well as the tests that are then conducted to help patients adhere to these guidelines. I'd like now to share with you my experience, both as a clinical researcher and a practitioner, to give you a sense of the territory and the navigation that is required.

CHOLESTEROL

The history of cholesterol-lowering drugs offers a particularly interesting case study. I was personally involved with numerous RCTs investigating the chronic condition of atherosclerosis. The studies lasted from a year to over half a decade. Scientific exploration had given rise to the lipid hypothesis, the idea that cholesterol was a chief culprit in hardening the arteries, leading to heart attacks, strokes, and peripheral vascular disease. The development of lipid lowering agents, targeting low-density lipoprotein (LDL) specifically, became an obsession of the pharmaceutical industry, and RCTs were the perfect tool for determining the efficacy of an agent.

The first point to make is that lowering cholesterol is only important if it leads to less morbidity and mortality for the patient. If family members of a deceased patient were told that he died with a low cholesterol level, that would be of little comfort. The endpoints of less angina, and fewer heart attacks, strokes, and death are ultimately more important. Cholesterol lowering is basically a surrogate marker for cardiovascular disease, meaning that a decreased cholesterol level in itself does not absolutely translate into fewer cardiovascular events. While decreased mortality from cardiovascular disease (CVD) is commonly found, Dr. Dubroff presents a group of forty-four RCTs that showed no decrease in overall mortality. The implication is that mortality was increased in some other area, perhaps due to the medication.

While lowering LDL is a well-established rationale for the prevention and treatment of CVD, at one point HDL was also studied intensively. Epidemiological and case studies had strongly suggested that HDL has protective effects. Yet, when pharmaceutical agents were created that significantly increased HDL and moderately decreased LDL, no reduction in CV events was found in high-risk patients. It is now generally accepted that HDL should lose the label of "good cholesterol." The problem illustrated here is that the development of cardiovascular disease is a multifactorial, dynamic process. We try to use different markers to develop a plan, but ultimately, we must keep our eye on the outcome. If not, polypharmacy, with its focus on managing various markers, will cause us to lose sight of the patients themselves.

More information can lead to more clarity as well as more confusion. Companies intent on marketing their drug end up conducting studies to show how statins decrease CVD in cases where the disease does not yet exist—for asymptomatic individuals—as well as for populations, including minorities and women, where they would like to expand their market. The Jupiter study by Astra Zeneca was undertaken to show that subjects without evident cardiovascular disease and normal cholesterol levels would benefit from lipid-lowering medications. But were these "healthy" individuals? A preselection criterium was having an elevated CRP, an inflammatory marker that is associated with increased cardiovascular events. Astra Zeneca used this marker to get a population with greater risk of the disease even as it was wanting to tout the benefits of the drug for people in general. The question becomes, when do we treat patients with statins as a preventative? Do we focus on those with an elevated marker for inflammation? Who is normal, and how abnormal does someone need to be to be treated prophylactically?

To assist the physician and patient in making an informed decision regarding when to start a medication, clinical guidelines have been instituted. The RCT literature is reviewed by preeminent experts in the field, and a consensus of opinions is presented. Of course, most lipid experts do consulting with the pharmaceutical industry, incurring conflicts of interest, but the bold attempt to provide a cogent picture of lipid management is still worthwhile. It is important to note that guidelines are continually updated as more studies appear. In 2013, the guidelines suggested that once you started statins, there was no need to do follow-up lipid testing. While the RCTs tracked levels, the idea was that once the benefit was established, the regimen was set. Not unsurprisingly, many doctors felt uncomfortable with not keeping records of changing LDL levels. Hence, the 2018 update reverted to testing to determine if adding more non-statin medications might help.

While a greater number of studies does not always lead to more prescribing, it usually does. Over time, the guidelines for those with cardiovascular disease have increased the pool of patients advised to take statins. The LDL level went from <130 mg% to <100 mg% to <70 mg%, depending on CVD risk factors. In Western society, LDL above 70 mg% is very likely. And the list of disorders that qualify as risk factors has increased dramatically. If you have diabetes, you will almost invariably fit the criterion for statin therapy. Note that the risk calculators are probably overestimating cardiovascular risk by as much as twofold as one ages and therefore exaggerate the importance of lipid management for patients over 75.

An important question is the degree to which outcomes are improved. Generally, for every 40 mg/dl% decrease in LDL, there is a

21% reduced risk of a major vascular event. Perhaps statins reduce CV risk through other means besides the lowering of lipids, by controlling inflammation, for example (unconnected to infection—cardiac trials involving antibiotic use were able to rule that out). And while drugs like Lipitor succeed in decreasing cardiac events, there is still a significant residual risk. Atherosclerosis is a complex process that cannot be managed by just one approach. Smoking is well-recognized as an independent risk factor, and in many cases, quitting smoking may be the most practical and beneficial course of action of all. Then, there is stress, which is hard to define and measure. Reducing stress via various methods is undoubtedly helpful, but the effects are hard to quantify.

In general, the narrow focus of RCTs on specific drugs to reduce specific markers can create a distorted picture for the doctor and patient who may fixate on the question of whether or not to prescribe a certain drug and completely lose sight of other options whose benefits may far outweigh the drug's benefits: lifestyle changes in the realms of diet, herbs, exercise, and emotional health. At the very least, they must consider the drug to be just one part of the picture. Corporations focus on using RCTs to prove their particular statin superior to the others, and one can find oneself focusing on the statistical difference between different agents while losing sight of entirely different avenues of exploration. Also, the medicine's practical value to the patient may be minimal and even negative when side-effects come into play. In all cases, there are risks, including an increased chance of becoming diabetic. Statins can also cause muscle ache and maybe muscle mitochondrial dysfunction. Even if the results are positive for prevention, do we necessarily want to treat someone for the rest of their lives with a medication that will prevent a disease that is not there?

Admittedly, the guidelines do recommend that the patient make an individual decision with their doctor. But the message is clear—more medications will lead to a healthier life. While lifestyle and diet are acknowledged to be part of the regimen, they are never given their due. RCTs are powerful tools, but they promote medication at the expense of lifestyle changes. Note that several groups that review the guidelines of the ACC/AHA do not automatically accept all the recommendations, even as they're working with the same data. The American Association of Family Practitioners, for example, divides the guidelines into three categories: will endorse, will not endorse, and something in between: "the guideline does not meet the requirements for full endorsement…but provides some benefit for family physicians." In general, doctors whose goal is the well-being of their patients and not the prescribing of medicine per se, should be wary of the elevated status of randomized clinical trials and do all they can to keep the bigger picture in mind.

HYPERTENSION

Hypertension is another interesting area of study because RCTs have turned its treatment into a colossal industry. Until recently, hypertension was not actively treated. When Franklin D. Roosevelt died of a hypertensive stroke in 1945, he had a systolic blood pressure of 300, rarely seen these days.

Part of the problem was the measurement of blood pressure. The noninvasive measurement of blood pressure (BP) using a cuff was only achieved in the early twentieth century. Moreover, before rigorous studies could be launched, the variation of blood pressure with time of day, activities, and psychological state needed to be addressed, as well as technical considerations such as cuff size, posture, and arm position. A BP reading can fluctuate easily during an office visit and often more than one BP reading needs to be done to determine a base for comparison. I was involved in many hypertensive medication trials, and it was extremely difficult but necessary to find stable patients for these studies.

Not until the 1960s were major RCTs executed to generate information that could be translated into guidelines. The Veterans Administration conducted crucial studies that were terminated early because of the significant difference between the medicated and placebo groups. It is interesting to note that they were following diastolic BP as the marker. Later, it would be realized that diastolic BP decreases as one ages while systolic BP rises, and eventually the latter would be considered the more important marker. But for a long time, there was rigorous debate about their relative importance. There are countless examples such as this of how science, and its "truth," is constantly evolving.

By 1977, the first Joint National Committee Report was instituted for the detection, evaluation, and treatment of hypertension. Thresholds for treatment were established, starting with the diastolic but progressing to the systolic, with the treatment threshold eventually becoming 140/90. As with the treatment of cholesterol, lower and lower levels were considered high risk, requiring more antihypertensive medication, particularly in combinations. There was always a nod to lifestyle changes and the importance of decreased stress, increased exercise, and a well-balanced diet to address obesity, but no means of attaining these goals was ever offered. There were no studies comparing a successful lifestyle program to the use of pharmaceuticals. Helping patients take responsibility for their health is difficult compared to giving them medications, and the results are hard to measure and treat in a rigorous scientific manner. A medication is a medication, easily quantified and standardized, but wellness measures are not. As we saw in the case of cholesterol, RCTs are designed to promote pharmaceuticals rather than patient selfcare, and guidelines have created a pharmaceutical bonanza.

The number of RCTs multiplied quickly as pharmaceutical companies vied to increase market share for their product. The federal government was actively involved in trying to sort out the advantages and disadvantages of different antihypertensives, individually and in combination. From 1994 to 2002, the National Heart, Lung, and Blood Institute supported a massive study to compare the effects of three different classes of antihypertensives and a diuretic. Involving 42,000 subjects from 600 clinics, the ALLHAT study lasted five years. Patients who started on one medication were able to add other agents, as they would in a clinical practice setting. The study was trying to mimic a true-life scenario, but as a result, its scientific validity was compromised. A more rigorous RCT might have provided more solid information, but then it would have had little to say about the reality doctors face in their offices.

In general, the narrower and more limited an RCT is, the more likely the findings are to withstand criticism, but the less likely they are to be applicable to a general population. All one can say with certainty is that the results apply to the given subjects in the study. The ALLHAT study attempted to be broader but for this reason it is, according to the standards of RCTs, vulnerable to criticism, and this is important to keep in mind since the study was used to establish guidelines. There were no clear winners, and the study was only about different pharmaceutical outcomes, not about the best overall approach for the patient.

In 2004, the National Heart, Lung, and Blood Institute appeared to put the brakes on treating hypertension by instituting a category of prehypertensives—those with a systolic blood pressure of 120 to 139 or a diastolic blood pressure of 80 to 89—advocating for this group lifestyle modifications rather than medications. This approach ended with the publication of the National Institute of Health 2015 SPRINT study, which suggested treating patients with levels as low as 130, if not 120. But the findings were mixed. While heart failure decreased with a lower blood pressure, heart attacks did not, and moreover, diuretics—and not lower blood pressure—could have been responsible for the results. Also, the usual finding of increased strokes with higher blood pressure was not found. Finally, many of the subjects had already been on antihypertensives when they entered the study; they could have been exposed to an increased blood pressure environment for many years and should not be compared to patients with new diagnoses. Altogether, to consider this study a major milestone in determining the treatment parameters for antihypertensives is suspect. Also, to adopt these findings would require the public to increase their intake of multiple agent antihypertensives, with a concomitant rise in side effects. As an example, 40% of the adult population in their 50s would be prescribed the drugs. The doctor and patient must compare the benefit of aggressive treatment with the drawbacks of various side effects, such as low potassium, hypotension, and fainting.

Big studies are supposed to lead to major advancement in treatment guidelines, but they can add to the confusion. Another National Institute of Health sponsored study, the ACCORD, found no significant reduction of cardiovascular events for diabetics whose systolic BP was lowered to less than 140, but did find a decrease in strokes (which were excluded in the SPRINT study). These findings were consistent with other antihypertensive studies. However, to achieve the decrease in strokes, adverse medication results more than doubled.

These studies represent just a tiny sample of the RCTs performed for cardiovascular amelioration, but they give you a sense of the process and evaluation of RCTs. Scientists could argue about my selection and my interpretations, but the overall point is clear: while RCTs have revolutionized medicine and given it more credibility, they have clear limitations on various fronts. And the answer is not simply the promulgation of more studies. Of crucial importance is the doctor and patient's wisdom in interpreting the studies, evaluating benefits, and including in their assessment all of the variables that affect a patient's well-being.

DIABETES

The bulk of my experience as a physician is with the study and treatment of diabetes, and this field provides an especially fascinating view of RCTs. The value of their scientific contribution is undeniable, and at the same time, it is very clear that RCTs are not the endpoint of good diabetic management.

The modern response to diabetes owes much to scientific and technological development on every front—diagnosis, management, and treatment. To begin with, the evolution of the monitoring of diabetes has been dramatic during my professional career. When I first started in the late 1970s, the patient would test their urine to evaluate their sugar control. This approach established a very gross approximation of diabetic health. At a given moment, a urine sugar could be high while the blood sugar was normal. Measurements of 24-hour urine glucoses would give some information regarding more long-term control, but the results could vary dramatically, depending on the patient's diet and lifestyle on a particular day.

A few years later, home blood sugar testing became a reality. The fingertip was pricked to get a drop of blood that was put on a strip and inserted into a Glucometer that would respond a minute later with a sugar level. Gradually, the meters became smaller and quicker, requiring less blood and providing results within seconds. Also, more painless means of obtaining blood with spring-loaded injectors and finer needles were developed. The result was that patients could take greater charge of their health and improve their blood sugar control by monitoring for themselves how lifestyle decisions were influencing their well-being.

In the last twenty years, blood sugar monitoring technology has continued to evolve at a fast pace. I was involved in an extraordinary number of clinical trials evaluating devices for the precision of their blood sugar readings as well as ease of administration. Because the glucose level in the interstitial space of the skin equilibrates with glucose in the bloodstream, continuous glucose monitoring can now be achieved bloodlessly with a tiny sensor inserted under the skin in the arm or the belly. The results can then be sent to different devices including smartphones. The ups and downs of blood sugars depending on diet, exercise, and stress can now be monitored in exquisite detail. Diabetics not on insulin do not need this amount of detail for good control. For Type 1 diabetics, however, it is a game changer. New means of measurement continue to be investigated, including methods that are one hundred percent non-invasive, such as shining ultraviolet light on the skin.

Another major advance in the field has been the long-term determination of good sugar control with hemoglobin A1c testing. The HbA1c test measures the amount of blood sugar attached to hemoglobin, the oxygen-carrying part of the blood cell. Blood sugars vary for many reasons, including diet, exercise, hormonal status, and stress, but this test is a reflection of the average blood sugar over three months (because that's how long a red blood cell lives) and positively correlates with diabetic complications over many years. It is a very dynamic number that can deliver a report card on the health status of the diabetic patient (though I performed a study at the end of my practice to show that the test is not infallible—more on this later).

A federally funded National Institute of Health study of Type 1 diabetes, the DCCT (Diabetes Complication and Control Trial) masterfully demonstrated the importance of good blood sugar control to decrease diabetic complications of the eyes, kidneys, and nerves. Over ten years (1983–1993), this RCT showed that lowering the HbA1c from 9 to 7 led to almost half the number of complications. The impressiveness of this study cannot be overemphasized. It adhered to all the principles of a well-done study, from appropriate recruiting to retention of patients. Plus, it was executed over an unusually long time-interval. The only drawback was that the bar of diabetic care was set so high that it would often be impossible to attain comparable results in the real world of medical care. But at least we know what is possible, and it provides a guiding light for doctors.

In addition to advances in monitoring, new means of delivering insulin have been introduced, hopefully leading to more physiologic control and ease of administration for the patients. The aim of newer technologies is not that they be more potent in lowering blood sugars but that they prevent hypoglycemia and help maintain blood sugars within a narrower range, reducing the seesaw of blood sugar changes. The holy grail is to implement a system of blood sugar control that is equal to the body's inherent homeostatic mechanisms.

Over the years, delivery systems have changed dramatically from reusable sterilized syringes (a major pain) to disposable syringes to preloaded insulin pens to pumps that continually give insulin in a variable, controlled manner. Now, there are closed loop systems where the pump can talk with embedded continuous glucose sensors to eliminate many of the daily manipulations of diabetic care. It is, however, a lot of paraphernalia for the patient to handle and not for everyone. Moreover, the cost can become prohibitive.

It is also important to note that increasingly sophisticated approaches do not necessarily lead to better outcomes. In 2019, a three-year study in the Czech Republic yielded surprising results. The researchers investigated continuous blood sugar monitoring versus frequent finger blood sugar testing as well as insulin administration from multiple injections versus continuous insulin administration by pump. Continuous monitoring of blood sugars improved HbA1c results dramatically, regardless of the delivery system. But using a pump with multiple blood sugar testing did much worse than multiple injections with continuous blood sugar testing. Apparently, the method of monitoring blood sugars was more important than the mode of insulin administration. It appeared that the more advanced insulin delivery system did not perform better, and there was even a trend that showed it not doing as well. The findings also suggest that the more information the patient is given, the more successful the outcome. As I am writing, more studies are being conducted of closed loop systems, which will almost definitely be superior to older insulin management systems. Nonetheless, it is clear that getting patients involved in their care and not just depending on technology is essential.

Overall, the advances have been extraordinary. In addition to developments in monitoring and delivery, the number of treatment options has exploded. Insulin was first extracted from the pancreases of cows and pigs in the 1920s by Banting and Best in Toronto. To their credit, they did not take out a patent, and injected insulin became a relatively cheap medication. Over time, different types of insulin products were introduced, with varying time courses of onset, peak effect, and duration. Science contributed to the industrialization of insulin with the introduction of the human gene into E. coli bacteria, producing unlimited amounts of insulin. Unfortunately, in part due to the need for meticulous RCTs to prove efficacy and differentiate between competing pharmaceutical products, the cost of this life-saving medication skyrocketed from a low of around $30 per vial (lasting about a month) to as much as ten times that price.

Once pharmaceuticals have been released, side effects can be most thoroughly monitored via large databases, a common practice in Europe. It appeared that a popular insulin product, Lantus, was showing increased cancer risk in some European databases but not in others. Those findings are ten years old, and no new data has revealed issues.

Type 2—non-insulin dependent diabetes—comprises the vast number of patients with diabetes, and here, the course of optimum treatment with medications is less certain. While the role of lifestyle is important in Type 1, in Type 2 it can be curative, without requiring any medication at all. So when Orinase, the first blockbuster Type 2 medication, came out in the 1960s, the question was raised as to its benefit. At the time, it was being dispensed without any formal RCTs having been done.

This deficit was addressed by an ambitious study by the University Group Diabetes Program. Unfortunately, after five years, there was evidence of excess cardiovascular deaths in the Orinase arm. A brouhaha erupted, and the trial was terminated for ethical reasons. But there was a major schism of opinion on the validity of the findings. Just a difference of three patients with a cardiovascular demise led to the significant findings. Moreover, the study was not designed to make any definitive statements about heart attacks related to treatment. The patients had not been randomized to eliminate the possibility of an imbalance in heart disease. In fact, there was, from the start, an excess of cardiac patients in the Orinase group. (This important procedural problem will be brought up later in this section as well as in the osteoporosis chapter.)

There were patients who were outraged that Orinase might be taken off the formulary when it had been so helpful to them and they'd had no serious adverse effects. Many physicians were befuddled as experts in the field took diametrically opposed stances. Upjohn, the pharmaceutical giant, argued that analysis problems led to potentially false conclusions while the National Institute of Health used the study to justify restricting Orinase use, though they did not ban it. As always, science does not lead to perfect conclusions, and RCTs with unexpected results can lead to major turf wars. The kerfuffle lasted for years with no clear resolution. Eventually, Orinase became obsolete, and thus the debate ended.

New classes of medications for treating Type 2 have emerged, making it difficult to determine the best way to proceed with any given patient. Diversity is good but adds complexity and cost. Big pharmaceutical companies perform numerous RCTs to demonstrate the superiority of their agent compared to others and to reveal short-comings with the products of their competitors. These studies aren't meant to converge on a single answer. For a doctor navigating the science, the territory is fraught with competing interests and divergent results.

A classic example is the meta-analysis of Avandia (rosiglitazone) and cardiovascular risk. Both rosiglitazone and pioglitazone are TZDs (thiazolidinediones—a mouthful to say), pharmacologic agents that increase insulin sensitivity and lower blood sugar. So how does one determine which agent is better? Insulin resistance had been determined to accelerate the atherosclerotic process, and thus these medications should improve cardiovascular outcomes. But when a meta-analysis review was done by Dr. Nissen, focusing on Avandia, he observed increased negative CV outcomes. The pharmaceutical company—GlaxoSmithKline—criticized the study, as did a host of respected diabetologists. Probably the biggest problem with the Avandia meta-analysis was that almost all the studies used had not specified CV outcomes as one of the outcomes to be examined (just as cardiac death was not listed as an outcome in the UGDP but became quite a controversy). Studies with no CV events were eliminated from the analysis, and questions were raised regarding the accuracy of methods used to determine CV events. There was also the problem of study heterogeneity since the enrolled diabetics had different degrees of CV risk. In general, meta-analyses are to be handled with caution since their conclusions depend on what studies are included and are vulnerable to basis. The various studies really are not comparable, having been designed with differing criteria and populations. Regardless of the lack of consensus regarding the meta-analysis, the negative publicity had a devastating effect on the sale of Avandia. Meanwhile, GSK did a three-year interim analysis (the RECORD study) specifically designed to determine Avandia CV risk, and none was found, but, of course, the controversy continued.

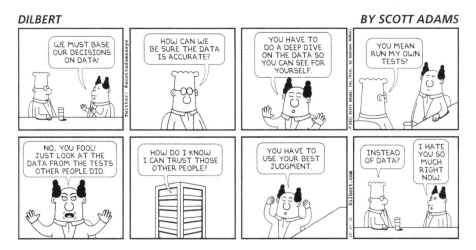

I would like now to talk about an RCT of my own that was meant to reveal the fallibility of HbA1c guidelines and the folly of blindly adhering to any set of standardized guidelines generated by RCTs. The gold standard test for determining the status of diabetic patients is the HbA1c, as already discussed.

It became apparent that during my years of practice, I had accumulated a cohort of unusual diabetic patients. In my group of anomalous patients, finger stick blood sugar testing (testing a variable number of times each day and recording results) showed good average blood sugar results while their HbA1c indicated poor control. Clinically, all sorts of problems need to be addressed regarding this conflict of data. The number one issue, unfortunately, is the honesty of the patients recording their blood sugars since people will either outrightly or unconsciously lie about their results. Perhaps they wish to please the doctor or want only good results to be recorded. Also, the blood sugar testing might have been done inconsistently and sometimes infrequently. Was I seeing a true representation of my patients' blood sugars during a twenty-four-hour period? It is a difficult question, but, having followed these patients for years and monitored their levels, I understood that I was in fact seeing an anomalous HbA1c finding.

The simple RCT that I set up in my office was to have the anomalous group compared to a comparator group that had in my judgment congruent HbA1c findings, i.e., consistent with expectations. For every anomalous patient entered, I enrolled a patient with an identical HbA1c that had the blood sugar results normally associated with that HbA1c. This pairing was done on a historical basis. At the beginning of the study, a baseline HbA1c was done to be compared to a reading after three months. I required all my patients to record all blood sugars in a book that I provided and that contained a daily grid for easy input of info, giving me the ability to review observational, longitudinal data. They tested their blood sugar before every meal and at bedtime and submitted their data every month to our office. (I had no funds to do more robust testing, such as continuous glucose monitoring.) HbA1c can vary so it was uncertain how the baseline groups would compare with this initial parameter. Amazingly, the two groups were identical with their average HbA1c results to start. There were approximately fifteen participants in each group, and they needed to submit at least 80% of all finger stick blood sugars to qualify for analysis of data. Despite the HbA1c being similar, analysis of the finger stick blood sugars showed the expected disparity. The recorded blood sugars were in the expected range in the comparator group, but the anomalous group had significantly lower blood sugars despite the textbooks' claim that high HbA1c levels show poor control. The test can be affected by mutations in an individual's hemoglobin that are genetic or caused by certain anemias; these individuals may have worrisome results while, in reality, they're doing well.

There were other parts to this study that I will not go into. All the information was handled by a University of Washington endocrine fellow who was managed by a full professor, Dr. Irl Hirsch. Admittedly, this study was not very sophisticated and, as with many studies, could be criticized in its execution and design. I had not a priori performed any analysis for statistical power. That would have told me how big a sample population I would need for a positive finding to be significant. Proving subtle differences requires larger sample sizes. It seems that my small-sized study just barely passed muster—the results were deemed statistically significant as soon as the last person was included in the analysis! HbA1c data in the anomalous group suggested a need for greater diabetic control while the finger stick results revealed no need for lowering blood sugars further. In fact, doing so might have led to significant hypoglycemia.

Nonetheless, the study reconfirmed a long-term observation of mine, and it was nice to have my clinical acumen substantiated. Also, it was a warning against blindly following HbA1c findings to determine blood sugar control and treatment decisions. Medicare deemed this test incontrovertible and considered the data it yielded the sole measure of success. Bonuses to doctors were to be meted out accordingly. While the standard may apply to a group, it may be inappropriate for the individual, and yet the doctor is pressured into applying it and, in cases where the desired level is not achieved, the doctor has no incentive to continue with that patient. Thus, "difficult" patients may find it harder to get consistent care. Furthermore, if a physician increases medication to lower blood sugar because of a high HbA1c without perusing finger-stick data, the results are potentially disastrous, with increased risks of hypoglycemia. I'm reminded of what teachers face when they are judged according to the test results of their students. Many of them feel that if they teach to the test, they will adversely affect the learning of their students. Similarly, doctors striving for an arbitrary HbA1c could damage the health of their patients.

Diabetes in the case of pregnancy is a good example of a situation requiring individualized care. Rigorous blood monitoring for the administration of insulin is more important than ever to avoid malformation of the baby, high birth weight with higher-risk delivery, and hypoglycemia for the baby. One of my patients was a young woman who was willing to do all she could to control her blood sugar. Insulin pumps were new, cutting-edge technology, and it was difficult to get insurance to cover it, but, knowing how important her specific needs were as an expectant mother and how capable and motivated she was,

I jumped through all the entangled hoops of the insurance company's procedures to get approval.

I also had to think creatively when caring for two diabetics who were morbidly obese when they became pregnant. These women were not insulin-deficient but insulin-resistant. They required massive amounts of insulin to lower blood sugars since pregnancy is an insulin-resistant state. One patient set a record of requiring 800 units of insulin per day, a challenge both logistical and financial, as regards insurance. Generally, 200 units would have been high, and over 400 units per day was almost unheard of, but the findings were clear and significant enough to present at a University of Washington conference on high-risk diabetic pregnancy. Yet again, we see how essential it is that every patient be seen as an individual and not a number or statistic.

ESTROGEN

The scientific study of female hormone therapy has been a roller coaster ride of benefits versus risks. There are three main uses for estrogen—symptom relief, birth control, and prevention of medical disorders for those with low estrogen. In the 1960s, estrogen was used for symptomatic relief of vasomotor symptoms, for hot flashes, and for mood stabilization. The most common preparation came from the urine of pregnant mares—Premarin. This was a "natural" product, but the preparation was definitely barbaric since the mare was pregnant with a foal that was considered expendable. Women did not know the manufacturing process but only the positive effects of counteracting menopausal symptoms. In the 1980s, unopposed estrogen use in women with intact uteri was associated with an increased risk of uterine cancer. Then, with the introduction of progestins to lower uterine cancer risk, estrogen use was once more in vogue.

Symptom relief is always desirable, of course, but one must always consider potential side-effects and evaluate the risk-benefit ratio. In the case of estrogens, the dilemma is dramatic and has spawned a good deal of questionable information regarding the best estrogen replacement treatment. Bioidentical hormone treatments are sometimes compounded, but this combination of different estrogens has, scientifically speaking, no proven benefits. In general, there are no well-done, large RCTs, only some small studies and basic lab studies demonstrating the different physiologic properties of different bioidentical hormones. Sometimes I feel that the dictum "To each, their own" is acceptable as long as negative effects are well publicized so that women can make their own decisions.

As an endocrinologist, I was regularly asked by women to ascribe symptoms they were having to hormonal imbalance that could then be alleviated by some type of estrogen therapy. I would always remind myself, "Do no harm." There were estrogen preparations, such as patches, less likely to lead to blood clots and cardiac events because they avoided the first-phase phenomenon of going through the liver. I was also careful with my diagnoses. Factors besides hormones can be the real issue, including the psycho-emotional environment.

Oral contraception began in the 1960s and has diversified into a host of hormonal combinations and delivery systems with greater ease of use and decreased side effects. The need for reproducibility of product, precision of dosing, and mass production required Big Pharma to get involved. The value for women as well as society was, of course, momentous. There is a slight risk of breast cancer and thromboembolic disease with hormone contraception use but decreased risk of uterine and ovarian cancer. The general perception is that the benefits markedly outweigh the risks for a large cohort of women. Black box warnings of potential problems are conspicuously displayed. For the individual patient, science does not offer definitive answers, but it has made possible the development of products that are extremely important to the well-being of women while offering some clarity about the risks.

In the past, estrogen replacement therapy was also widely accepted. Observational epidemiological studies revealed that the incidence of coronary heart disease among women started to climb after menopause. The obvious implication was that the decline in female reproductive hormones was the cause and that maintaining a premenopausal estrogen status could be beneficial. Then came the Women's Health Initiative (WHI) study in 2002, an ambitious, primary prevention trial of coronary artery disease and breast cancer with the use of postmenopausal estrogen. A total of 16,608 women with an intact uterus were given Prempro, and more than 10,000 hysterectomized women were given Premarin. There were two other arms of the study that did not use hormones but rather a low-fat diet or calcium-vitamin supplementation as comparison.

Unfortunately, there was a 50% dropout rate during the study that affected the robustness of the conclusions. And the study has been criticized since the average age of the women was 63, which is 10 years postmenopausal, with 26% having preexistent heart disease. The Prempro arm was stopped after five years because interim results suggested increased risk of coronary artery disease, stroke, and pulmonary embolism. The Premarin arm did not show any increased coronary heart disease risk and even showed a decreased risk. Also, there was protection from breast cancer. But this arm was also terminated early because of the increased incidence of blood clots.

The increased risks became well-publicized, and hormone replacement therapy plummeted. But was this warranted? The study does not prove that estrogen in general is the problem. Perhaps, it is oral estrogens specifically that cause clots since they pass through the liver; estrogen patches that absorb through the skin avoid this problem. Possibly, the estrogen combined with progesterone was more the problem than estrogen by itself. Or perhaps the issue could be traced back to the use of mare's urine. A separate line of inquiry concerned itself not with the deaths that estrogen might be causing but the deaths potentially prevented by estrogen use. In 2013, a mathematical analysis of WHI data titled "The Mortality Toll of Estrogen Avoidance" attributed 18,600–91,600 hypothetical excess deaths to the lack of estrogen replacement therapy. The paper emphasizes its cardioprotective power, the prevention of osteoporosis, and the relief of menopausal symptoms. At the same time, the findings suggest that postmenopausal estrogen use does not increase the risk of breast cancer. This phenomenon was confined to the combined estrogen-progestin arm, and the use of alternative progestins has since been shown to eliminate that worrisome finding.

The problem with the WHI study was the way the public reacted to the findings, causing many women to reject estrogen replacement even when it could have been beneficial. I particularly remember discussing estrogen replacement with women who had breast cancer. While they were very symptomatic with severe hot flashes and increased emotional lability, they remained unwilling to use even transdermal estrogen to alleviate their suffering. It was hard for them to look at the data and evaluate the risks and benefits in a dispassionate matter. And no wonder, when the discussion had veered between extremes, estrogen being considered lethal on the one hand and protective on the other. There is no straight path from scientific observation to medical practice. Instead, there are multiple, divergent paths to consider. The experts argue, and the poor patient is left in the middle wondering what to do.

OSTEOPOROSIS

Let us delve into a relatively new area of medical interest and concern, namely osteoporosis. Until recently, most women were not living long enough to develop osteoporosis. But now, better medical and obstetrical care has increased the number of years women live in menopause, an estrogen-deficient state, with vertebral fractures, loss of height, and dowager humps. Female hormonal replacement had been central to maintaining bone health, but the treatment of osteoporosis really took off once bone mineral density, or BMD, could be easily measured. Intensive study established the levels of BMD that lead to significant increases in fractures, particularly for the hip and spine, and Big Pharma began the search for new medications.

Thus began the development of bisphosphonates. In 1995, a study of alendronate by Merck showed a 48% reduction in new vertebral fractures compared to a placebo over a three-year period. It is important to realize, however, that this finding is a relative risk reduction. You might be told that a medication will halve your risk, but if your risk for fracture was only 6% to begin with, then in absolute terms, the reduction will be 3%. Clearly, how the data is presented affects the discussion of pros and cons. If the reduction is only 3% (and in general, subsequent medications have had similar outcomes), you might not be as interested in starting a medication, perhaps for life, with various potential side-effects, including atypical fractures.

Overall, a 3% decrease in fractures can make a lot of economic sense and lead to a healthier society, but how do we assess the treatment options for the individual? The Fracture Risk Assessment tool, or FRAX score, was developed to help individuals determine their personal risk and the ten-year probabilities of having a fracture. It takes into account additional factors—personal and family history of fractures, current smoking, corticosteroid use, and rheumatoid arthritis. A comparison is made with age-related individuals of the same gender. In the end, a score is generated and compared to the guidelines. The recommendation is that a 20% chance of vertebral fracture or a 3% chance of hip fracture over a ten year period of time warrants treatment in women.

A major downside of this assessment is that it does not take falls into consideration since this data was considered unreliable and not analyzable. That's extremely unfortunate because 95% of all hip fractures are related to a fall and the majority of spinal fractures are related to car accidents, with the rest caused by falls, sports, or acts of violence. There are many studies that examine ways to decrease falls via yoga, tai chi, hip protectors, etc. In some individuals, these practices may be far more helpful than medication. Lifestyle changes should always be of primary importance, but we live in a culture that often looks for quick fixes and eschews patient responsibility. Big Pharma provides solutions that minimize the need for patient involvement.

The thought is: "I take this medication, and I'm good to go." But it is not that easy.

Fluoride, which prevents dental caries, looked like a good candidate for increasing BMD and decreasing the fracture rate. In 1990, a trial with 135 women over four years showed a tremendous increase in BMD—35% increase in the lumbar spine and 12% in the femoral neck, compared to 9% in the lumbar spine and 6% in the femoral neck for alendronate. These are extraordinary numbers, and yet at the same time, there was a significant increase in fractures. Apparently, increasing BMD does not necessarily lead to fewer fractures. Issues of bone quality versus quantity become an important consideration. In the end, the goal is to avoid fractures. While BMD defines who is osteoporotic, it is not itself the cause of fractures but merely a surrogate marker.

Strontium, a natural mineral, enhances the process of building bones by stimulating bone-building cells while at the same time decreasing bone reabsorption. Bisphosphonates work only on the latter. Algaecal is a product containing strontium as citrate, sold in the United States as a supplement for bone health. Strontium increases BMD by being a heavier cation than calcium, and thus when strontium replaces calcium in the bone, it will increase the BMD, but this will not necessarily lead to stronger bones. That can only be determined by data on fracture rates, preferably in an RCT setting. Clearly, boasting that Algaecal is good for bone health because it increases the BMD is not a sufficient reason for its use. But no one will do the additional studies for economic reasons. Supplements do not have the return on investment to justify costly RCTs.

However, in Europe, they did do the appropriate study with strontium combined with ranelate, not citrate. Strontium ranelate was the proprietary compound of a small company in Europe, sold under the name Protelos. In the United States, while strontium citrate was classified as a supplement and could be sold over the counter, Protelos would have to be submitted for approval by the FDA as a pharmacologic agent, which the small pharmaceutical company was not prepared to do. Two studies of the compound by the European Union

(SOTI and TROPOS) showed a reduction in fracture risk comparable to that produced by the pharmaceutical drugs. Not only is strontium ranelate a less expensive product, but also its dual action is a plus. In the initial studies, there was no mention of any serious adverse events, but in 2012, a strontium ranelate study that was designed to demonstrate the efficacy of Protelos in males suggested a higher rate of cardiac events. The increased cardiac risk might be explained by an imbalance in the population since cardiac problems were not part of the randomization process. This is a problem we have seen before (see discussion of Orinase and Avandia in the section on diabetes). It runs counter to the design principles of RCTs to try to evaluate an uncontrolled finding or give it any significance. Good science would dictate new, well-controlled studies to properly examine cardiovascular risk. The Servier company decided to suspend Protelos for lack of financial resources to address this potential cardiac side effect. There have been several reviews of national databases, showing no increased cardiac risk or blood clots with strontium ranelate use. Denmark did a nationwide cohort study from 2005 to 2011 showing no increased risk of acute coronary syndrome. A retrospective cohort study in the United Kingdom showed no increased risk of blood clots with either strontium ranelate or bisphosphonates. None of these studies confirmed the adverse effects. Regardless, negative publicity in Europe and the cost of further study caused Servier to withdraw strontium ranelate. Later, in 2018, the Indian company Aristo put their version on the market, including a black label warning detailing potential adverse effects.

Clearly, science does not provide definitive answers. It is a cumulative process that involves ongoing interpretation and reevaluation. My personal experience navigating with my patients the science in a number of areas—cholesterol, hypertension, diabetes, estrogen, and osteoporosis—has taught me the importance of a sophisticated understanding of the science, both its language and its methods. Only then can we make best use of the data that we have. We can acknowledge its limits and dedicate ourselves to practicing the art of medicine alongside the science.

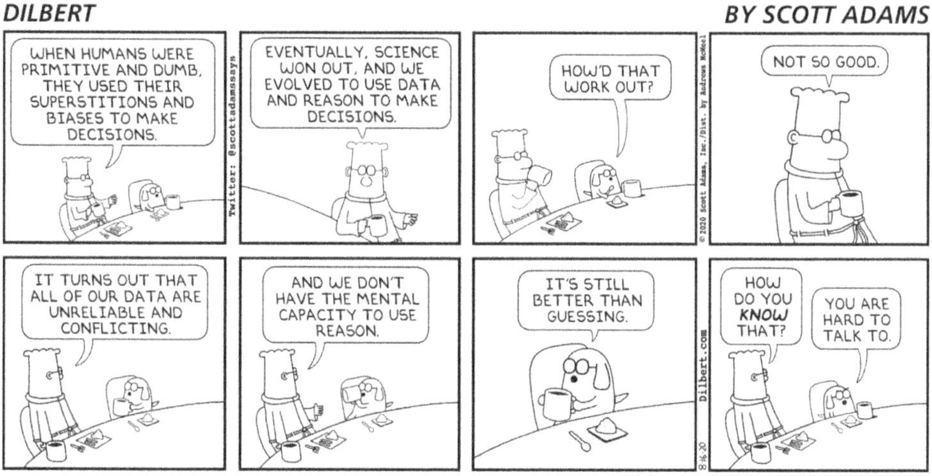
DILBERT
BY SCOTT ADAMS
WHEN HUMANS WERE PRIMITIVE AND DUMB, THEY USED THEIR SUPERSTITIONS AND BIASES TO MAKE DECISIONS.
EVENTUALLY, SCIENCE WON OUT, AND WE EVOLVED TO USE DATA AND REASON TO MAKE DECISIONS.
HOW'D THAT WORK OUT?
NOT SO GOOD.
IT TURNS OUT THAT ALL OF OUR DATA ARE UNRELIABLE AND CONFLICTING.
AND WE DON'T HAVE THE MENTAL CAPACITY TO USE REASON.
IT'S STILL BETTER THAN GUESSING.
HOW DO YOU KNOW THAT?
YOU ARE HARD TO TALK TO.
Twitter: @scottadamssays
Dilbert.com

CHAPTER FIVE

Expanding the Field: Alternative Medicine and Diet

As long as we think of medicine as predominately a science, we will focus on clinical trials. For the most part, these are conducted by the pharmaceutical industry and designed to promote the consumption of drugs. In truth, the field is so much richer, and there is so much for the practicing physician—and anyone interested in their health—to explore and understand. I would like, in the remainder of this book, to discuss other essential aspects of the healing art. These include integrating alternative medicine and lifestyle choices, cultivating a profound doctor-patient relationship, and acknowledging and harnessing the power of mind and spirit.

The treatment of disease with drugs is just one approach to medicine, and it is shaped by a well-defined paradigm whose mantra is war on the invaders. A completely different approach is to embrace the positive forces of healing, to summon the body's own inner resources and, where there is dis-ease—understood essentially as a lack of ease, to bring the system as a whole back into balance. Consider the difference between antibiotics and vaccines. While antibiotics seek and destroy microbes by warfare, vaccines enhance the organism's immune system to prevent or nullify the action of invasive infectious agents. There is no war, just containment and disposal of unwanted intruders. The noxious substance is surrounded and made impotent and then eliminated naturally.

Science can be reductionistic, fragmenting the body into parts and examining how the parts fit together. The disease is isolated, and elimination is the goal. But what if the system as a whole becomes the focus? What if disease is seen as the outcome of a lack of connection within the whole? Francisco Varela said it well: "If a living system is suffering from ill health, the remedy is found by connecting with more of itself" (Levey & Levey, 2014, p.176). The focus is not on the damaging disease but on the living, thriving whole.

HERBAL REMEDIES

Allopathic medicine, while it supports vaccines, does not concern itself with stresses that throw the body out of balance. Usually, it waits for the full-blown disease to manifest in order to then treat it with medication and surgery. While it recognizes that stress kills because of dysregulation of the body, it does not recruit the body's natural ways of promoting well-being but instead imposes external treatments.

Naturopathy, while it does have similarities to allopathy, is of a more holistic bent, emphasizing natural medicines with less potency and fewer side-effects as well as diet modification. Herbs are used, often in combination, to recruit the healing powers of the body to bring the body back into balance. An example is a group of herbal products called adaptogens, meant to alleviate the stressed body from chemical, physical, or biological insult and thus return the body to homoeostasis. Ginseng for immune support and stress reduction and Ashwagandha for regulating metabolism and calming the brain are two examples of these medicaments, which are not recognized by allopathic medicine.

While herbal preparations are becoming more accepted by conventional medicine, they are still considered a secondary treatment option. We have seen how debatable the RCTs are in the case of pharmaceuticals, and still the drugs are approved. Non-pharmaceuticals such as strontium, on the other hand, have a more difficult time.

When there is a fear of risks, there are fewer resources for further study, and so the substance is banned for lack of counterbalancing evidence. Big Pharma encounters many difficulties in its design of RCTs, but they can throw more resources towards correcting shortcomings and promoting their products.

Let us explore the studies that have nonetheless been executed. Berberine, which is of interest to endocrinologists, was the subject of two different studies in China in 2008, both strongly suggestive of the therapeutic action of berberine. One study involved newly diagnosed Type 2 diabetics who were given either berberine or the drug metformin, an excellent first-choice medication for diabetes. Both groups improved equally over a thirteen-week course of treatment. Another study added berberine to an already prescribed treatment regimen and reported the benefits of this addition. The results were encouraging and appear to show at least equal efficacy compared to the drug. Unfortunately, the studies were small with fewer than fifty individuals and thus not definitive. And they would be torn apart for inadequate description of the berberine product, no blinding of the products, and in the case of the second study, the heterogeneity of the treatment group. For these reasons, science has rejected berberine as a viable alternative, even though berberine would most likely pass as a legitimate agent if a larger, well-controlled study were performed. Unfortunately, no resources were allocated to such a study.

As another example, let us consider the use of cranberry products for urinary tract infections (UTIs). In one high-quality study, conducted by Kevin Maki over a three-year period and involving 370 women with a recent history of UTIs, the daily consumption of eight ounces of Ocean Spray cranberry juice was compared to a placebo consisting of multiple substances that together tasted like cranberry juice. The results were 39 clinical UTIs in the treatment group and 67 in the placebo group. Meanwhile, basic science has worked out a rationale for the benefits, showing how cranberry interferes with the attachment of E. coli to the bladder wall and also suppresses inflammation resulting from bacterial infection. Is that enough justification for cranberry to be considered therapeutic for UTIs?

The Cochrane Collaboration, a global, independent, non-profit network of researchers, professionals, and patients, uses a rigorous set of criteria to scrutinize all available evidence. Regarding cranberry extract, it tells us that we cannot draw firm conclusions due to the heterogeneity of the various studies. At best, the conclusions have been tepidly in support of positive effects. The criticisms of many of the studies were small sample size, compliance issues, high dropout rates, and inadequate statistical power. On the other hand, cranberry products have been used by countless women who report benefits, suggesting that a well-designed RCT would have positive results. I have experienced the therapeutic effects of cranberry extract. For 48 hours, I dealt with the symptoms of a UTI with painful urination every hour, but I did not want to start an antibiotic until a urinary culture had been obtained. I decided to start cranberry extract and had very significant improvement in my symptoms. Let us just say that getting up just twice a night was a welcome relief. When the symptoms later recurred, they were once again alleviated with cranberry extract while I waited for the antibiotic. Just because the studies corroborating my experience do not meet every standard does not mean I'm going to dismiss cranberry as a treatment or avoid recommending it to patients. But the danger of the Cochrane Collaboration is that certain treatments will lose credibility. Their rigorous criteria are admirable, but it is a shame if nuggets of interest and useful treatment options are discarded because they cannot meet the tests designed for pharmaceutical agents.

Let us consider another review of the evidence supporting the use of herbal products. In Germany in 2017, there was a systematic review of herbal medicines for gastrointestinal disorders in children and adolescents. A wide net was cast, starting with 10,083 abstracts, but 9,824 were immediately excluded because they did not involve RCTs, were not written in German or English, or did not include children. In the end, fourteen studies fulfilled the criteria. This list still contained possible deficiencies of bias due to randomization procedures, inadequate blinding of participants and personnel, and data and reporting deficiencies. Nonetheless, the conclusions of the systematic review were that "an emerging evidence base for the use of certain herbal medicines for conditions such as diarrhea, dehydration, infantile colic, IBS, and functional abdominal pain" was demonstrated.

Herbal medicine is generally accepted in other parts of the world. During a trip to India, I became ill, suffering from a sharp pain under my tongue that I eventually diagnosed as oral herpes. My throat was so swollen that for three to four days I took almost no food or drink. Physicians who were among my fellow travelers provided me with an antiviral as well as lidocaine, but I continued to be extremely debilitated from not being able to swallow. I had previously visited the Tibetan medicine museum and had the chance to chat with the curator about the process of making herbal preparations. I went back to see her, and she took me over to the Tibetan medicine clinic to see one of their physicians. He spoke English, but the exam was cursory. He took my pulse, blood pressure, and examined my tongue in what seemed a perfunctory way, making no attempt to locate my supposed lingual ulcer. Clearly, his diagnostic system was completely different from the American allopathic one. The pronouncement was a hot liver, and generally being hot. His treatment plan included a list of foods that I could and could not have. Then, he wrote prescriptions for three different herbal preparation pellets. Also, an external balm was ordered that I could apply to my neck to relieve my extreme throat discomfort. The balm was very helpful and dramatically improved my ability to swallow almost immediately. I took the herbal preparations for about four days until I felt 90% better. So far, I have not been able to determine which herbal preparations I was given, but the experience made me a believer.

HOMEOPATHY

Naturopathy and the use of herbs is just one of the alternatives to allopathic, drug-centered medicine. Another, homeopathy, has had extraordinarily little legitimacy in the general medical community because it is based on principles that are unfathomable to the scientific mind. Herbs have well-described mechanisms of action and have often been used by pharmacologists to produce medications, but homeopathy is speaking a different language entirely. Basically, the "active" substance is diluted using alcohol or distilled water until it is reduced to such a degree (less than Avogadro's number) that it is theoretically no longer present. Then, the preparation is vigorously shaken in a process called succussion. The conundrum is how to study the effect of something when it is unlikely to be materially present.

The important distinction to make in evaluating the field of homeopathy is between the theory and the practice. Many discussions that I have read summarily reject homeopathy because of difficulty with the theory, and so there is no consideration given to its actual effectiveness. Since the system does not fit with an overall worldview, it is rejected automatically.

While there is a dearth of rigorous studies, six systematic reviews have been performed. The results of these meta-analyses are not stellar, but small, specific effects do appear to be present, separating homeopathic treatment from placebo. There are different practices of homeopathy that also need to be addressed. An individualized approach appears to lead to more positive results. Placebo effects may be involved in these cases since spending over an hour with a patient to determine a treatment plan affects the clinical outcome. The individualized approach also makes it difficult to evaluate homeopathy since patients with the same issue will be given different treatments. The heterogeneity of treatments and outcomes, along with the difficulty of maintaining an impersonal approach to the healthcare visit, does not allow for objective scientific analysis. The systematic reviews identify all these deficiencies, leaving us with about twenty studies of uncertain bias, none completely clean. Of course, many pharmacology studies, as we have seen, have their biases and deficiencies. At this point, no decisive conclusions can be made about the efficacy of homeopathy, but that does not mean that there is no evidence. What is needed is a way to conduct and evaluate studies, whether within the RCT realm or otherwise.

ACUPUNCTURE

Acupuncture is another example of a belief system foreign to the allopathic mind, but it has a 5000-year history—plenty of time to discover what techniques actually work. It is based on a holistic energy system, and treatments attempt to bring the system back into balance. It is effective for many conditions and has proven beneficial by evidence-based studies. The Acupuncture Evidence Project has done a systematic review of over a thousand studies. With meticulous care, they present the evidence, with as high a quality of proof as any medical study, for allergic rhinitis, chemotherapy-induced nausea and vomiting, low back pain, knee osteoarthritis, migraine or tension headaches, and postoperative pain. Their conclusion is that "it is no longer possible to say that the effectiveness of acupuncture can be attributed to the placebo effect or that it is useful only for musculoskeletal pain" (McDonald, 2017, p.55).

For other conditions, including hypertension, insomnia, irritable bowel, anxiety, schizophrenia, asthma, anesthesia, and multiple types of pain, there is compelling evidence, but it does not meet the highest scientific standards of acceptance. Standard criteria for evaluating evidence-based studies are difficult to apply. For example, how can one establish an appropriate control group alongside the active needled group? Should the placebo group have needles inserted in a supposed non-therapeutic area or pressure applied in a therapeutic area without the insertion of a needle?

As for the theory, it makes little sense from a Western perspective. Terms such as a hot or cold liver, indecipherable in the realm of allopathic medicine, do not refer to the physical organ or its temperature. Therapy is performed along meridians of the body that have never been physically identified in an autopsy. Since acupuncture was developed before the establishment of the scientific method, you could speculate that while the practitioners made valid observations, they did not have the means nor tools to develop an appropriate theory explaining these observations. In any case, our lack of understanding should by no means lead us to reject a clearly efficacious therapy.

COMPLEMENTARY AND ALTERNATIVE MEDICINE

I am comfortable with ignorance, and a fear of the unknown is not going to prevent me from exploring this and other alternatives to allopathic medicine. I was pleased to participate in a workgroup for the integration of complementary and alternative medicine (CAM), established by the Washington State Insurance Commissioner. A Washington State bill in the late 1990s required insurers to include "every category of provider" in their plan. The insurers wanted to know how to determine what practices would provide true health benefits to the patient, and CAM providers wanted financial support on a par with that received by the conventional healthcare industry. Over a period of three years, each CAM specialty had the opportunity to present their system of practice.

The most impressive group, in my mind, was the midwifery group, whose schema mapped out in great detail their operations. They integrated allopathic obstetrics with a powerful emphasis on the relationship between the pregnant woman and her midwife. They promoted home birthing as opposed to institutional environments to maximize the emotional well-being of the woman. There was never any over-reaching of midwives to deliver babies in high-risk situations. Limitations of the practice were well-recognized, and good working relationships with obstetricians and hospitals were cultivated to ensure a safe delivery. Midwifery worked in partnership with allopathic practice in such a way that the best of both was achieved.

The physically interactive alternative therapies were represented by chiropractic and massage therapy. In these areas, it is virtually impossible to use RCTs to verify efficacy independent of strong placebo effects. Blinding the practitioner is impossible since they need to know what they are doing at all times! Chiropractors, however, have a long history of being utilized in labor and industrial injury treatments, so a great deal of data is available to evaluate outcomes and financial benefits to employers. In their presentation, the practitioners never addressed the underlying theory of subluxation (the misalignment of vertebrae). Practical results were enough.

In the end, a voluminous report was submitted. It did not offer definitive conclusions and could not create immediate change, but the whole three-year process established a basis for change. It led to the formation of crucial, new relationships—among insurers, conventional providers, and CAM providers— and interdisciplinary dialogue was established to a degree unheard of previously. Many of the key issues were identified and discussed, and agendas for further work and research identified. For example, there was a clear need to do more research to establish clinical efficacy of CAM procedures and cost effectiveness.

In my own practice, I had the opportunity to integrate alternative therapies at my community hospital, holding for two years the title of Director of Alternative Medicine Services. Small and medium-sized projects were pursued with the assistance of a health administrator. The health club added classes on meditation, Qi Gong, and yoga to broaden the options for rehabbing patients. The psych unit transformed a small outside area into a working garden for patients. And I opened a hospital-based herbal pharmacy. We hired a consultant to give lectures on the benefits of herbal remedies to generate interest among the staff and give them a knowledge base.

The biggest problem with using herbal products is the variability of the potency and purity of the medicinal plants. Our consultant chose high quality brands to be stocked. A feng shui environment was created for the outpatient pharmacy to further enhance therapeutic effects. The intention was good, but the results were not. I am not sure why this experiment failed, but it might have been a combination of the high cost of high-quality products and the lack of a dedicated pharmacy staff to guide the patients. National surveys suggest that almost 20% of the population use herbal medicine, but our hospital's attempt to link herbal medicine with the allopathic system was not successful. Still, some of the small projects that were started during my term as director are ongoing. In the wellness center, yoga has become mainstream. The integration of conventional with alternative medicine is a long process, and minor successes must be savored.

DIET

Diet has always been an important part of my conversations with patients, and no one doubts its effects on health. But with the studies of diet, as with all studies, whether of drugs or alternative therapies, there are the usual issues with collecting unbiased information, dealing with confounding variables, and drawing generalizable conclusions.

In any study of diet, the food consumed must be meticulously recorded. Studies using data recall, however, have obvious problems. A study of food intake by scientists (supposedly a group of highly objective, detail-oriented individuals) revealed that food recall for the previous twenty-four hours was highly inaccurate. Reported food intake was underestimated in some studies of obesity by half. In RCTs, the accuracy of food data can be enhanced by using the AMPM (USDA Automated Multiple-Pass Method), which is very labor and time-intensive and does not work well for a large, long-term study. The process is so intensive that it might drive some participants to indulge in food or drink simply for comfort and relief.

One of the main thrusts of a randomized study is to eliminate confounding issues. In nutritional studies, this is particularly hard to do since food has very strong personal and cultural characteristics. Different populations eat differently, and their food preferences are inseparable from their lifestyles. Also, the media plays a big role in how people eat, promulgating diets that lower cardiovascular risk, cancer incidence, and inflammation. There is so much information flying about that you can find a proponent for any food or diet you like. We're also lectured about all the foods we must avoid. Speaking tongue in cheek, I would tell my patients that for any food they're interested in, they are bound to find a study proving it to be unhealthy. Only cardboard will be exempt.

For millennia, diet has been recognized by many cultures as critical to maintaining health and treating diseases and disorders. Ayurvedic medicine is particularly focused on shaping diet according to individual psychological and physical characteristics. There are three constitutional types called *doshas—vata* (air + ether), *pitta* (fire + water), and *kapha* (water + earth). Specific foods are prescribed for different body types—a truly holistic approach.

Meanwhile, in Western culture, there has not till recently been the same degree of attention to diet. In fact, the upper classes have tended towards debauchery. The most influential person on diet in the twentieth century, Ancel Keys, noticed that well-fed business executives had high rates of cardiovascular disease while the rates were much lower among the common folks in the Mediterranean area. Reviewing diet information, he concluded that animal fats were an incriminating factor. In the 1960s, he performed a massive observational study to show the benefit of olive oil, vegetables, fruits, low-fat dairy products as well as pasta, rice, and potatoes. His Seven Countries Study demonstrated a connection between the Mediterranean diet and decreased cholesterol levels and cardiac deaths. However, he did not address the issue of low occurrence of heart disease in regions with high-fat diets, such as Denmark, France, and Norway, or the fact that Chile has a high incidence of cardiac disease with a low-fat diet. The complex issue of trying to study the effect of diet independent of the psychosocial environment is daunting.

A large, randomized study exploring the benefits of the Mediterranean Diet (PREDIMED) was performed in Spain with results published in 2013. It was a valiant effort and received many accolades for being a well-designed, rigorous study in a real-world setting. There were three groups—a low-fat control group and two Mediterranean diet groups, consuming either extra virgin olive oil or a combination of nuts. Participants based their meals around vegetables and fruits, legumes and whole grains, and avoided saturated fats and sweets. Fish or seafood were eaten at least twice a week. They were allowed to have a glass of wine every day but no red meat, only white. Unfortunately, the low-fat diet arm of the study was unsuccessful in changing the eating habits of its participants, so theirs was a "modern" diet including red meat, sodas, and commercial baked goods.

The initial population was highly diverse. They did not have overt cardiac disease but had a high risk of it, with either diabetes or some combination of smoking, high LDL, low HDL, obesity, or family history of premature cardiac disease. Half of the subjects were on lipid-lowering agents. The diabetics could be on oral agents or insulin, and half of hypertensives were on antihypertensives. Hopefully, the randomization process would equalize this diverse group of treated individuals so that the results would be meaningful. The beauty of a rich, variegated population is that it better reflects the world we live in, but as noted earlier, it is less "scientific." The good news is that the study demonstrated a decrease of 30% in cardiovascular disease events and a 49% reduction in strokes from the Mediterranean diet. Some problematical randomization procedures, however, required a reevaluation of the conclusions, and there was no consensus as to their validity. With all the potential noise in the data and confounding factors, it is remarkable that the study has received such acclaim. From a scientific point of view, this study comes closest to passing scientific muster, but we can make no general claims for the efficacy of the Mediterranean diet. It is not like a statin benefit that can be clearly scrutinized.

Another study, the touted Lyon Heart Study, is vulnerable to the same criticism since it is hard to isolate which elements of the diet were important for the statistically significant decrease in heart attacks. Moreover, the diet of the control subjects was not monitored during the study for fear that any monitoring might influence what they ate. Only at the end of the study were the diets of the controls and the experimental group compared, and there were the usual problems with fallibility of dietary recall.

The diet study that I feel best demonstrates the reduction of cardiac risk was actually more of a lifestyle study, lasting five years. The protocol, designed by Dean Ornish at Stanford, included a diet that was a lot more restrictive than any Mediterranean diet—a 10% fat, whole foods vegetarian diet—along with extensive monitoring and support for exercise, stress management, and group psychosocial work. The study required a tremendous number of resources and was very labor intensive. In addition, only a very select group of subjects was willing to submit to such a strict lifestyle regimen. In the end, there were only 48 patients with documented coronary artery disease enrolled. Nonetheless, the results were impressive, with more than twice as many cardiac events in the control group. Remarkably, there was even some regression in the stenosis (blockage) of coronary arteries in the experimental group while there was increased stenosis in the control group. The study's significance lies in its emphasis on the need to go beyond diet in order to maximize improvement. While this approach may be unrealistic for many people, for those who are willing, the benefits are clear.

Often, the benefit of foods goes unstudied. Who will pay for the rigorous study of garlic, for example? At the same time, certain food groups can be marketed just like pharmaceutical agents, and there is plenty of incentive to mischaracterize and mislead. For decades, the sugar industry has funded distinguished scientists' work downplaying the role of sugar in heart disease and promoting an expanded role for carbs. The main message was that red meats with their saturated fats were detrimental to your health, with only a slight nod to the positive health effects of polyunsaturated fats. Fruits and vegetables, being low in fat, were said to provide good carbohydrates, but there was little attention given to the importance of their fiber content. The result was an increase in refined carb use that led to a significant increase in the incidence of obesity and diabetes. One of the main problems is that carbs are sweet, and we consume too much for increased gratification. Even artificial sweeteners have their critics, who claim that they increase appetite and consumption, causing changes in the microbiome and glucose dysregulation.

At the other extreme is the low-carb paleo diet. The rationale for this diet is that in Paleolithic times, hunter gatherers ate meat, berries, nuts, vegetables, and fruit—a high protein, high fiber, low carb diet. In the last 10,000 years, agriculture has changed our eating habits. The paleo diet has not been studied like the Mediterranean diet, so to give more heft to this meat-centric diet, a meta-analysis was performed on studies looking at red meat consumption and cardiovascular risk. The conclusions were that there was a low to very low amount of evidence that reducing unprocessed red meat intake would reduce the risk of cardiovascular mortality and stroke. The studies that were used for this review were selected based on GRADE (Grades of Recommendation Assessment, Development and Evaluation), which is a system that examines the validity of RCTs. GRADE is not considered helpful in evaluating observational studies, which would include most dietary studies. The Lyon Diet Heart Study, for example, did not qualify. Completely discarding the information in that study and others with similar conclusions leads to a biased outcome. To make matters worse, the lead author is part of a Nutritional Recommendation Consortium that has a partnership with Texas A&M, which gets funding from AgriLife—an organization that promotes Texas beef. Earlier, it was the sugar industry that skewed our ideas. Clearly, data can be finagled to bolster opposing claims on any dietary issue.

The amount of information on the benefits of various diets and foods continues to grow exponentially. Given the clear shortcomings of any study, I would be circumspect regarding any eating plan that severely restricts a particular food group. Moreover, too many shoulds and should nots lead to anxiety and stress far exceeding the benefits of any program. There is a term for becoming too fanatic with diet information: orthorexia, an obsession with eating healthy foods and completely avoiding others that are thought harmful. The physician plays an important role in working with a patient towards an individualized program of health and wellness that is neither idiosyncratic nor overly stressful. If the studies teach us anything, it's that moderation should be its defining quality.

PEARLS BEFORE SWINE   **BY STEPHAN PASTIS**

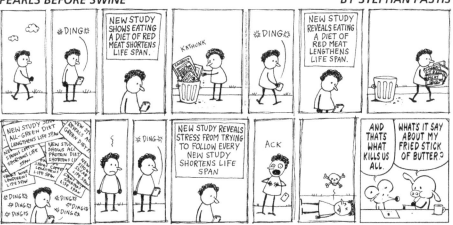

THE ART

"The possession of knowledge does not kill the sense of wonder and mystery. There is always more mystery."

Anaïs Nin

THE ART

"The possession of knowledge does not kill the sense of wonder and mystery. There is always more mystery."

Anaïs Nin

CHAPTER SIX

Cultivating Relationships

Practice in the field taught me that being a doctor is not just about applying the science that is taught in medical school. It is about building connection. To do so successfully and wholeheartedly requires cultivating one's humanity, in particular the qualities of humility, compassion, and respect. It is a unique journey for every physician, one that is potentially profound.

ACKNOWLEDGING BIAS

Sherlock Holmes, in "The Adventure of the Cardboard Box," famously says in answer to Watson's wonderment, "We approached the case, you remember, with an absolutely blank mind, which is always an advantage. We had formed no theories. We were simply there to observe and to draw inferences from our observations." It is an admirable ideal and the goal of every scientist, but how often are we able to be absolutely rational in this way?

In the medical field, as we have seen, science can only take us so far. Studies are subject to bias, both in their design and their interpretation. Moreover, doctors who have to apply the science they learned in medical school to real-life scenarios are likewise vulnerable to bias. It is essential that doctors acknowledge this reality. They can then cultivate a practice of observing their own thoughts and emotions. They may notice when these are less than rational and actively interfering with the accuracy of their observations and analysis.

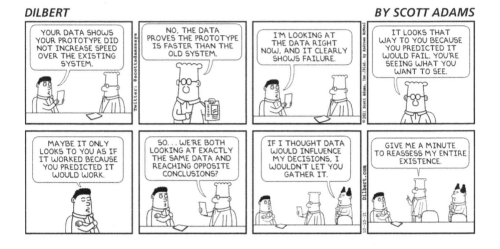

Thoreau observed in his journal on January 5, 1860, that "a man receives only what he is ready to receive… The phenomenon or fact that cannot in any wise be linked with the rest which he has observed, he does not observe" (Thoreau, 1984). It simply does not exist. "If it is spoken, we hear it not, if it is written, we read it not, or if we read it, it does not detain us." An experiment designed by psychologists Christopher Chablis and Daniel Simons provides astonishing proof of Thoreau's insight. Participants were asked to watch a video in which two teams had each been given a ball to pass among themselves. They were told to count the number of times the players on the team with white shirts passed the ball. After they gave their answers, they were asked whether they'd noticed the man in the gorilla suit wending his way through the crowd of players, stopping to pound his chest before exiting. More than half hadn't, and they were astonished when they re-watched the video and saw the gorilla clearly. He was obvious in his big, hairy suit, but since they were so intensely focused on something else, he'd become invisible.

How often are people blind to what they consider extraneous? "We miss more by not seeing than not knowing," said the great Dr. Osler

(Epstein, 2017, p.19). Consider the scientifically rigorous RCTs. Part of what makes them rigorous is their clear definition of goals and outcomes. Only a clear definition allows us to design the study properly, making sure that it is randomized so that the final outcome is not skewed by the population selected. The question is, in our desire to measure specific outcomes, and in the narrowness of our focus, what may we be ignoring? Things that may later come to seem incredibly obvious? And how often do doctors, in their focus on medical facts and treatment protocols, lose sight of the patients themselves?

Then, there are the errors that doctors are vulnerable to when they must come up with diagnoses. The psychologist Daniel Kahneman describes the various cognitive errors that prevent us from making dispassionate evaluations. The priming effect refers to how we are prejudiced by what we have already been exposed to. Kahneman instructed a group of subjects to chat about foods and then later asked them to fill in the missing letter in SO_P. You probably know which letter they were more likely to choose, whether A or U. A doctor who has just identified a virus in one patient is that much more likely to assume that the next patient suffers from the same ailment. Confirmation bias has to do with our desire to confirm preconceived concepts or ideas. Often, a doctor will stop looking for more information as soon as there is evidence confirming the beliefs he or she already holds.

Then, there are heuristics—simple rules which people use to form judgments and make decisions more efficiently. These mental shortcuts usually involve focusing on one aspect of a complex problem and ignoring others. We need these shortcuts so we can bring our decision-making to a conclusion and proceed with a plan of action. In the medical field, the possible diagnoses are too many to count, so doctors, in order to rule out possibilities, are encouraged to focus on the more likely. "When you hear hoofbeats, don't think of zebras" is a well-worn aphorism. The story of Occam's razor is evoked to argue for the solution that is simplest, requiring the fewest conditions. Unfortunately, these approaches can stifle curiosity and disguise the complexity of a situation where individual human beings are involved. There is no obvious answer to this problem except for doctors to be aware that it exists. They can strive to be as thorough and careful as possible in their gathering of information, and for this reason, clear communication with patients is essential. Encouraging patients to be aware of their own biases is also helpful.

In the interest of cultivating self-awareness, let me illustrate some of the more common short-cuts that occur in the decision-making process. One is the judgment heuristic. Consider, for example, a well-dressed businessman who enters the clinic with shakes, sweats, and tremors. It would be easy to assume that he is suffering from some sort of virus while giving no consideration to the possibility of heroin drug withdrawal. The affect heuristic has to do with how our emotions influence decisions. Perhaps a doctor is pained by the number of patients who have died from a particular condition and is therefore emotionally attached to the idea of having all patients tested for that condition.

As a practicing physician, I have often witnessed these heuristics at work. At one point, a patient came to me with a diagnosis of low potassium. The problem was that the MD had ordered a whole blood potassium test and not corrected for a relatively low normal red cell count. Potassium is basically found in the red cells, and the fewer red cells, the less potassium. Correcting the potassium result for the red blood cell mass led to a normal result. At the same time, I noticed that her symptoms and history were consistent with stress and depression. When I tried to explain to her that her potassium was in fact normal, she became irate and said her doctor would never have sent her if that were the case. She stormed out of the office, and several days later I received a letter from her physician demanding to know how I could contradict his findings. The doctor was too attached to his diagnosis and unwilling to examine his biases. Perhaps the availability bias—"if it comes to mind, it must be important"—was at play, as well as confirmation bias—he may have seen low-potassium patients with similar symptoms. These biases are human frailties and will occur even with well-informed physicians. What is needed is a willingness to change course.

Another example from my personal experience involves a man in his sixties, admitted to the hospital with an irregular, fast heart rate. The patient had a history of cardiac disease and was now experiencing mild heart failure. The cardiologist, who was very learned and well-regarded, was having trouble lowering the heart rate, and routine testing, which included thyroid tests, indicated thyrotoxicosis. The cardiologist consulted me, convinced that the patient was suffering from thyroid storm, and was amazed when I started treating the patient for thyrotoxicosis rather than thyroid storm, which is a very specific diagnosis associated with temperatures usually above 104. The doctor could not let go of the more ominous diagnosis, even though he'd received the specialized input of an endocrinologist and even though textbooks disagreed with his labelling. He went ahead and prescribed steroids, which were entirely unwarranted. The patient was not sick enough to undergo dubious therapeutic treatments, but the doctor was in the grip of availability and confirmation biases and afraid the patient would destabilize. Of course, we all want to avoid terrible outcomes. The challenge is to prevent our fear from clouding our decision-making.

Sometimes the error in judgment is so egregious that it justifies a legal case. I described one of these earlier, the case of the young man who died of advanced diabetic ketoacidosis. The patient was seen very cursorily, the first time with no lab done and no consideration given to his weight loss, increased urination, and profound weakness. The physician could well have been exhibiting cognitive ease (not thinking very hard), judgment heuristic (here was a young male with no history of chronic illness, so one is less likely to think he had any comorbidities that needed to be addressed), and availability heuristic (the doctor had seen a lot of respiratory illnesses in the previous days).

I have coined the term, Expert Paradox, to deal with another kind of bias. Physicians who are extremely well-versed in a particular field may find it challenging to look for answers in areas where they are not conversant. They will focus on what exists in the realm of their expertise. Thus, the most knowledgeable and sophisticated physician may be the wrong doctor to see with a hard-to-define illness. Overall, my point is that there is no science without interpretation or bias. Probably, the most important quality for a physician to have is humility. Science does not provide us with all the answers; plus, we will make mistakes. It is good to aspire to objectivity, but to ignore our subjectivity is unwise and will ultimately hurt our patients.

As long as we think of medicine as predominately a science, we will be working with the assumption that the doctor, rigorously trained in certain sciences—anatomy, chemistry, etc.—will have all the answers. But the doctor is human, and so is the patient. Medicine is an art because humanity lies at the heart of it. Recognizing our humanity will allow us, both as doctors and patients, to be aware of our frailties and inspire us to delve into areas that lie beyond the scope of science—the cultivation of self-awareness and human relationship.

COMMUNICATION AND COLLABORATION

At the heart of medicine is the relationship between doctor and patient. I cannot emphasize this enough. Being taught the science, knowing the facts, and coming up with a diagnosis can only take a doctor so far. In collaboration with the patient, the doctor must define what constitutes good health and the goals of care. In almost every situation, there is complex territory to be navigated, requiring on the part of the doctor flexibility, humility, and the ability to listen.

My most meaningful interactions took place when I connected with my patient as a human being, and together we tried to understand what was happening and what would help. While the system wants to standardize, every patient should be individualized. The doctor must learn about the patient's view as regards technology versus naturalism, maximal versus minimal treatment, and belief versus skepticism. There are many questions to be discussed. Every day, new technologies emerge, but when are leading-edge developments crucial to the cure? Often too much is done for little reason, or people think newer is better. How far one goes in exploring the possibilities is determined by the proclivities of both doctor and patient. Decision-making in the face of uncertain, inaccurate, and imperfect information is a challenge, and both parties can be guilty of investigating the options too much or too little. Sometimes, the final decision can be to do nothing at all, just wait and see.

Certainly, "slow" medicine has its virtues. I was referred a 92-year-old man after a neck CT scan, ordered for other reasons, revealed that he had a thyroid nodule. I was somewhat hesitant to do a thyroid aspirate since it wasn't clear that we would proceed with surgery even if the results came back suspicious for cancer. Also, more than 20% of the pathology results end up being indeterminate. Nonetheless, I did the thyroid aspirate, and the path report was definitive for a papillary thyroid cancer, which is often cured by surgical removal of the thyroid.

Now comes the melding of the art and science of medicine. The fact is that papillary thyroid cancer tends to grow very slowly, and there are documented cases of patients doing well for many years without surgery. At the same time, papillary cancer tends to be more aggressive in the elderly. For a 92-year-old patient who has lived a long life, it is uncertain how much benefit will be derived from trying to prolong his life, especially when complications from the surgery may shorten it.

I sat down with the patient and his son and explained the diagnosis and the uncertainties surrounding surgical removal. They listened attentively and came to a firm decision. Instead of immediate surgery, we would monitor the growth of the tumor, and if the growth appeared aggressive, surgery could be entertained. Remember, before the CT scan was done, there were no concerns at all about a thyroid mass; it was an incidental discovery, for which we have a term: incidentaloma. I respected the calm and thoughtfulness that went into their decision-making process, which was remarkably free of anxiety. The last time I saw the patient was two years later, and there was no evidence of significant growth of the cancer. The incidentaloma did indeed turn out to be incidental.

In general, many thyroid aspirate referrals are generated by incidental findings of inconsequential thyroid masses—the CTs and MRIs have been done for other reasons. But it is often hard to reason with a patient regarding the inutility of doing the aspirate and the value of adopting a wait-and-see attitude. Similarly, hard-to-feel nodules are seldom malignant, but because ultrasound has made it possible to aspirate these nodules, patients often prefer to proceed rather than live with not knowing.

Physicians can help their patients assess risk by presenting the data on risks versus benefits in a dispassionate and discerning manner. It is easy for the risks to become overblown. I saw this at close range when my own wife was pregnant. Routine blood testing in the first trimester was slightly abnormal, suggesting thyroid overactivity, and her OBGYN wanted to send her to an endocrinologist, especially since at the age of 38, she was already considered somewhat high-risk. I did not think it was necessary, however. Her weight was stable despite some nausea and vomiting. Her energy level was acceptable and pulse was normal, with no fine tremor of her hands. I also did a physical exam of her thyroid and noted nothing of great concern.

My experience and the literature both supported a wait-and-see approach, and in the end, it was a transient thyroid abnormality that resolved within six weeks. To have gone to a specialist would have caused my wife more stress and made her more aware of having a "high risk" pregnancy. Diffusing the thyroid issue into a "no rush" situation improved her general attitude and physical status. The OBGYN, clearly anxious about high-risk pregnancy, had been led by the affect heuristic.

Even as I always aimed for rational discussion of the data, in presenting my patients with the facts, I felt the need to acknowledge that medicine is permeated with uncertainties. Science itself admits that it must continually reexamine its conclusions, striving for a truth and objectivity that is not attainable, only approachable. A healthy skepticism, as long as it does not lead to paralysis, is good.

I've mentioned the critical importance of a holistic approach. Big Pharma focuses on drugs, but a person's health depends critically on lifestyle choices, such as diet, exercise, and psychological well-being, so as a doctor, I always included these in my analysis and discussion. Minimizing stress was always essential. When I would see a newly diagnosed Type 1 diabetic teenager with their mom, the first part of the visit would be dedicated to establishing a connection and tempering their anxiety and distress. Diabetes often conjured up all sorts of negative stereotypes, crushing the teenager's belief that they could lead a healthy, happy, and long life. My mantra was: "You've been given the opportunity to be healthier than your peers. By monitoring your blood sugars and learning what diet and activities help your body function best, you'll become that much more aware and actively engaged in leading a healthy lifestyle." Jokingly I might add, "Could the diagnosis of diabetes be the best thing that ever happened to you?"

Then, with patients whose control had deteriorated, our first consideration was not what other medications should be added or manipulated, but what could the patient do to bring the blood sugars back into balance? Not what had they done wrong, but what could they do right? Patients can lose their way because of stress or lack of activity. The winning prescription could be twenty minutes on an exercycle and using the sauna, rather than recriminations about how they got themselves into this mess and turning to pharmacology out of a sense of failure or hopelessness.

I learned a lot through my years of practice about the diversity of approaches that converge to create a successful healthcare encounter. Rather than adhering blindly to rules or preconceived plans, I preferred to engage with my patients as individuals, taking into account their habits, attitudes, and psychological well-being. Every conversation was unique, depending on the patient and their circumstances. There was never one answer, one size fits all. When it came to deciding a course of action—whether or not to do testing, undergo surgery, take medication, or make lifestyle changes, whether to act or do nothing at all—I preferred a holistic approach. It required ongoing communication and collaboration, and I found it to be that much more dynamic and gratifying and ultimately successful.

CARING, NOT JUST CURING

The healthcare system asks doctors to focus on the disease—to label the problem and then cure it so it no longer exists. However, this is only a part of the doctor's role, and it largely ignores the person who is suffering from the affliction. I have found the following distinction, made by Buddhist practitioners, very useful: *Pain is an affliction of the body while suffering is an affliction of the self.* Even when doctors cannot cure the body, there's still much they can do to alleviate their patients' suffering.

Some of my finest moments helping patients occurred when we weren't even talking about a specific medical issue. Over time, I got to know my patients, and they got to know me. Some patients would schedule a visit and tell me they needed to seek my counsel regarding their lives. I would act simply as an observer of their human frailty and strive to be present with them. I might not be effecting a cure, but I was still the person who was most familiar with their medical condition and could therefore serve as compassionate witness of their pain and suffering.

I still vividly remember a young woman who had insulin-dependent diabetes as well as a progressive, inherited, degenerative, neurological and cardiac disorder that left her wheelchair-bound and completely dependent on her caretaker. Since traveling to the office was a major undertaking for her, I asked her to come for annual visits only. Her caretaker was well-versed in diabetic management, and I simply found myself supporting their treatment regimen, offering very few suggestions or changes. We did conduct blood tests to monitor her diabetic status and the general functioning of her organs, but I always felt my most important job was to be a thoughtful, compassionate person in her life. We spent most of the visit discussing whatever topic the two of them cared to raise. Even though I could not effect a dramatic change in my patient's health picture, she and her caretaker always left the office happy and satisfied.

I find it hard to describe this young woman. She was so pure of heart, majestic, and radiant in the midst of her devastating physical dysfunction. On her chest, she sported a heart tattoo. She left me with the feeling that there was absolutely no need to feel sorry for her. And she made vividly clear the distinction between a person and her disease. There is the affliction and then there is how you live with it.

As doctors, we can realize that we are in a truly privileged position to help a patient to *be* with their affliction. This may seem counter to our goal of eliminating the affliction, but the two are not contradictory, and if we focus too narrowly on the cure, we forget this most important aspect of our patients' well-being. The truth is, while the doctor is focused on cures, the patient is looking for care.

It is useful at this point to distinguish between empathy and compassion. Empathy, a complex cognitive process that engages mirror neurons, allows a doctor to feel what the patient feels. Attenuating empathetic response may be very important in some healthcare situations where the healthcare provider is identifying too much with the pain and discomfort of the patient, diminishing the quality of their care. You do not, for example, want your surgeon to be overly concerned with the marring of your body from an incision. And it is important for healthcare providers to modulate their empathetic processes, so they do not damage their own mental health and get burned out. Compassion, on the other hand, is a different process and activates a part of the brain that is connected to prosocial motivations and reward mechanisms. A healthcare provider with compassion wants to approach, help, comfort, and alleviate suffering and can do so without incorporating the pain.

A patient of mine lived with severe rheumatoid arthritis for decades, undergoing intensive treatments. My role was simply to monitor her thyroid condition. I had tremendous admiration for her grit and determination in maintaining an active lifestyle that included wilderness hiking. Unfortunately, she developed an autonomic neuropathy that led to problems with heat stroke and chronic dizziness. Her increasing disability led to a bad fall, which required her to be admitted to a rehab center. Still, she did not want to change her lifestyle. When her various doctors, a neurologist, a cardiologist, and her long-term rheumatologist, could not solve her dilemma, she came to see me. We spent time talking about her symptoms, and I learned about the ways in which she had coped in the past. She had refused to be inhibited by her condition and continued to function at a high level. Now, however, she was realizing that the medical system could no longer support her in this endeavor. She welled up with tears and thanked me for listening with compassion to her story. Her focus shifted, and she was able to talk about finding ways to adjust to her evident limitations. No longer intent on a cure, she could begin to figure out how best to maintain her quality of life.

Toni Bernhard, an academic lawyer who developed a chronic fatigue disorder that played havoc with her life, wrote a book: *How To Be Sick*. No specific label could be given to her debilitating illness, nor was there any definitive treatment plan. She describes how she coped and learned to navigate a complex and often insensitive medical care system. Self-compassion became immensely important, along with a sense of equanimity regarding what she could and could not do. She was also able to express gratitude for all that she had accomplished in her life—raising children and pursuing a successful career. She was a meditator, and she liked to recite this verse from the Buddhist master Nyoshul Khen Rinpoche:

> Rest in natural great peace,
> This exhausted mind,
> Beaten helpless by karma and neurotic thought,
> Like the relentless fury of the pounding waves
> In the infinite ocean of samsara.

Bernhard was not able to fix her condition. Instead, she acknowledged the inevitability of her pain and suffering and heard through it all the invitation to "rest in natural great peace."

A woman in her twenties was referred to me for low potassium. She was poised, thin, and well-dressed, a successful professional. Her symptomology was nonspecific, basically malaise and tiredness, and she did not report any gastrointestinal problems, such as abdominal pain, nausea, vomiting, or diarrhea. Upon physical examination, the only remarkable findings were poor care of her teeth (slightly surprising because of her comely appearance otherwise) and small abrasions and calluses on her knuckles.

She appeared to be trustworthy, and I did not sense any subterfuge. But when I looked further—*Dr. Watson, the diagnosis is obvious!*—I realized she had bulimia and was using cathartics and vomiting to induce weight loss. When confronted with the diagnosis, she broke down, crying that she was worthless and her appearance disgusting. I comforted her, telling her that her low potassium would return to normal as soon as she stopped her vomiting and purging. She was obviously a very successful individual who needed to learn how to love her body. I told her that finding a good therapist was essential and that I'd be happy to keep seeing her for any physical problems. I wrote a letter to her doctor letting him know of her eating disorder and its likely effect on her potassium levels. She never returned to see me, hopefully because she and her primary care provider, now aware of the nature of her ailments, could look for the appropriate treatment.

The challenge is always to remain as open-minded as possible. One can never know where a visit may lead. Often, at the end of a first visit, I'd find myself discussing treatment plans that were unrelated to the initial reason for the visit. Many women would come in saying there was a problem with their hormones and ask me to fix it. They said they were "fine" regarding emotional or psychological stresses, but with enough discussion, as well as patience and caring, stories would emerge of significant psycho-emotional trauma, such as rape or sexual assault, events that the patient had never discussed with anyone, not even their psychiatrist. They would sometimes experience a catharsis and come to a better understanding of how these issues were affecting their health. This scenario took place often enough that my medical assistant would keep tissues at hand. And if the patient left tearful, she knew there had been a breakthrough of some sort.

"The secret of the care of the patient is in caring for the patient," wrote Dr. Francis Peabody at the beginning of the twentieth century (Peabody, 1927, p.877). More recently, Dr. Vivek Murthy, Surgeon General under Presidents Obama and Biden, argued that friendship is critical to promoting good health outcomes (Murthy, 2020). Dr. Bernie Siegel, a pediatric surgeon at Yale, makes the same argument in his amazing book, *Love, Medicine and Miracles.* "When we commit ourselves to egoless, unconditional love, true healing begins" (Siegel, 2002, p.8). These are the words of a skilled surgeon who fully understood the importance of serious medical intervention. But even as he administered chemotherapy with harsh side effects, Dr. Siegel advised his patients to perceive the chemicals, not as toxins to be feared, but as beneficial agents to be embraced. He saw love operating on every front.

Dr. Kathryn Montgomery advises more restraint. She suggests that doctors should act like good neighbors with their patients, rather than friends. In her opinion, an overly engaged doctor will have trouble with boundaries and lose the ability to be objective. I understand Montgomery's concerns, but in my over thirty years of practice, I experienced the overwhelming benefit of cultivating close, intimate relationships with my patients, of being their "friend." Emerson said that a friend is "a person with whom I may be sincere." Time and again, I saw how trust and authentic communication were critical to the successful outcome of a visit. I imagine that such trust and communion may even enhance healing because of the circulation of the hormone oxytocin, which is stimulated by compassion and care. In any case, I know that my deep engagement was often the lifeline that helped a patient get through an illness. It is easy for doctors to underestimate the impact of connecting with their patients if just sticking to the facts of the situation. But, in the words of Margaret Wheatley, "when we seek for connection, we restore the world to wholeness. Our seemingly separate lives become meaningful as we discover how truly necessary we are to each other" (Levey & Levey, 2014, p.235).

An insulin dependent diabetic patient whom I saw for over twenty years told me many times that without our emotional and physical aid, he would never have survived. I first saw him as a young teenager who received very little support from his adopted parents. In fact, I never even met them. The boy was basically alone in the world, and my medical assistant and I became his surrogate parents. After high school, he was absolutely on his own since his parents offered him no help at all. He did not have an easy life, his erratic blood sugar levels making it difficult for him to hold down a job. While he had Medicaid for insurance, he often did not have the resources to buy food. We would feed him and help him out with extra insulin and blood sugar testing supplies. He would work very hard trying to control his diabetes so he could stay employed—he did not want to be a burden on society. When he eventually got a girlfriend, he dedicated himself to being her devoted companion as well as surrogate father to her child. He had an exceptional ability to roll with the punches and, instead of complaining, maneuvered through life with a smile. I always admired his quiet nobility. We went through many trials over a twenty-year span, building a strong friendship based on honesty, care, and understanding.

It has always been important to me to see my patients as a whole, their psychological and physical well-being intertwined. The benefits of such an outlook were particularly clear in the case of a patient whom I initially saw for treatment of his cholesterol level, a very smart and successful aerospace engineer. He wanted to see a lipid specialist because he had a strong family history of cardiovascular disease, and testing had shown some evidence of atherosclerosis, or hardening of the arteries. Together, we reviewed the literature and decided on the most prudent course to take. He was an active person who did not show any symptoms of heart disease, but he was often depressed, and we discussed his life in detail, including his marriage, hobbies, and outlook on life. His problem could best be described as a pervasive sense of ennui. At one point, he mentioned his interest in photography and how he had given it up because it required him to travel when he did not have the time. He was never as engaged or lively as when he talked about the pictures he had taken, and I suggested to him that photography might be exactly what he needed to give his life meaning. He thanked me and left the office, planning to go on photo shoots around the United States. He entered photo contests and began to win awards, even as he continued his work as engineer. I attended his exhibitions, and he gifted me with his photos. He went so far as to credit me with saving his life by encouraging him to reengage with his passion. Studies have shown that adults with a higher purpose in life reduce their risk of death. *Eudaimonia*, which literally translates as "good spirit," is Aristotle's term for the flourishing of individuals when they pursue their highest potential. A doctor is specialized in what is good for the body, but this cannot be separated from the person's well-being as a whole.

There were various occasions when patients' issues had no medical answer and pursuing an endocrinologic workup would have been in vain. Often, the patient needed to look inwards as well as outwards, and the most I could do was support them in that process. As in other cases I've described, the success of the visit depended on my ability to listen. There was the case of a twenty-two-year-old woman who came in with her mother, wanting a hormonal workup to make sure that all was normal. She had been diagnosed since age ten with depression, and there was a history of depression on her mother's side. My discussion with her did not suggest any active depression at that time, however. Other family history problems weighed on her, such as migraines and the difficult-to-control hypertension that her brother had likely inherited. There were some symptoms that suggested PMS. She had successfully graduated from college in library science and had a job in a library but was not able to work regularly because of her illness.

I told her that I did not consider her problem to be endocrine-based, but that it was very important that she not doubt her symptoms and feelings. The fact that doctors could not identify a cause did not make her dis-ease less real. Perhaps eventually, a doctor would discover the issue, but in the meantime, she needed to cope with her problems, deciding what her limitations were, even if others could not understand or accept them. Then, the conversation went in an unexpected direction. I told her that her plight could have some positive features. She probably had gained some wisdom into the human condition and developed a sense of compassion for other people's struggles. She acknowledged her heightened empathy for others and then mentioned how difficult it must be for me to see such a "difficult" patient as herself. My response was that she was at that moment having more empathy for me than herself! At the end of the session, both she and her mother thanked me profusely for my attentiveness. In this case, my role had been to help my patient direct more positive thoughts towards her self-care, setting her on a path towards improved well-being.

In general, my practice was shaped by the profound belief that a problem is real, whether it is physical or psychological. If a patient is not feeling well, then this is the truth, and healing of some sort is in order. Often, the patient's healing did not require my expertise in endocrinology. What they needed was to reveal their physical and emotional pain and have their story be heard. I'm reminded of the movie *Intimate Strangers* by Patrice Leconte. A young woman with marital problems goes to see a psychiatrist but mistakenly walks into the office of a tax accountant. The receptionist knows that there is no appointment, but the woman is so sure that she is in the right place that she is ushered in. She's harried and does not give the accountant a chance to explain who he is. As a tax accountant, however, he is used to listening well, so he just sits there while the woman describes her distress. At the end, she feels satisfied that she has been heard and gets up, declaring she will be back the following week. Eventually, she learns her mistake but finds no reason to discontinue the visits.

It was my ability to be compassionate and patient that allowed me to take care of a patient who would otherwise have fallen through the cracks. This patient was a high-powered, driven guy who could be difficult to handle. He had had a pheochromocytoma, an unusual adrenal tumor, removed several years before I saw him. He came to me with nondescript pains in his abdomen. After nuclear imaging, it was determined that there was another tumor present at the site of the previous surgery. I had him operated at the University of Washington, and the tumor was successfully removed. There was no evidence of metastatic spread, but a year or so later, he developed nonspecific, depressive symptoms and scattered pains in his upper back and the back of his head. Extensive imaging revealed no tumors. Still, I believed there was a recurrent, metastatic tumor present and had him go to the Mayo

Clinic. None of their imaging tests found anything incriminating and, because of his difficult personality, they had a psychiatrist see him. They basically left him feeling that nothing was physically wrong with him. He came back irate and decided that he would see no other doctor but me since I believed his symptoms to be real. He was now requiring increased pain medication to control a host of worsening pains. I persuaded him that he needed to see other specialists. He eventually went to the National Institute of Health where they were able to find the elusive tumors. There was no treatment to cure him, but he was much better off when he knew he was not crazy and that his symptoms were real. Our relationship was close, and I believe he benefited tremendously from my faith in him and from a brotherly love that went beyond what most doctors would consider a part of their duties. In my experience, this love is intrinsic to the healing process.

I want to say something about the value of laughter. Laughter and humor are important coping mechanisms, helping to maintain equanimity during stressful, difficult decision-making times. Movies have been made about Dr. Patch Adams and his clownish approach to the practice of medicine. Physiologically, laughter can increase the release of endorphins in the brain and increase brain connectivity as well as social connectivity. A memorable, short documentary, *Laughter Yoga*, by Dr. Madan Kataria, describes his use of laughing yoga in the case of diagnoses such as cancer to decrease stress and promote a stronger immune system. It's more than a laughing matter. In my own practice, humor always played an important part and was appreciated by almost all my patients. My desire was always to turn the doctor's visit into a positive experience rather than a dreaded one.

PATIENT AUTONOMY

The virtues of patience and compassion became very clear in the case of a patient whom I got to know very well over the course of about fifteen years. He was diagnosed with diabetes as a child, and when

I first saw him, he was very sullen and withdrawn. His parents had divorced, and he had moved with his mother to Seattle. He was traumatized by his experience of medical care, having been hospitalized several times for life-threatening diabetic ketoacidosis. He was poked so often during these hospital stays that he developed an extreme antipathy to needles. He did acquiesce to injecting insulin but refused to do finger-stick blood monitoring. His diabetic control was not good, nor was it horrific. Every visit, I would bring up the need for him to start testing blood sugars to improve his diabetic control, and every time, he would refuse.

Now, here is a common issue, and I know of doctors who would reject patients who openly disobey doctor's orders and fail to adhere to a basic standard of care. The medical system, having become less and less understanding of the reality doctors face, blames them for a patient's decision not to test blood sugars and incentivizes getting rid of all such patients. From my perspective, however, I was looking at a patient who cared about taking care of himself but had a profound need for more personal control. I thought this need quite understandable, considering the chaos that life had dealt him. It is often quoted that Hippocrates said he'd "rather know what type of person has the disease than the disease." And so, though it might put a blemish next to my name, I decided to take the road of always being very attentive and present with him and not assault him with moral judgments on his decision not to test.

Through the years, we were able to get to know each other well. I continued to bring up the need to test blood sugars, but we could be lighthearted about it. He would come back for appointments and would even introduce the topic by saying he was still not testing. At the same time, I did think that it was important to address the issue each time. It never felt futile to me, and I never lost hope that change could happen. By at least working on a healthy diet, he was helping himself immensely, more than if he tested blood sugars and did not eat properly. Eventually, he found a job and got married. He continued to try to balance out diet, exercise, and the use of short-acting insulin. There were episodes of low blood sugar, but they were never incapacitating. Then, he had a child and came in beaming, not just because he was overjoyed at being a dad, but because he had also started testing his blood sugars! He could not test blood sugars for his own sake or his wife's, but he could do it for his child. What a stellar example of the fact that we never can know what the ultimate outcome will be. This case, as so many others, was an inspiring confirmation of the importance of patience, humility, and faith in every person's potential.

In general, my practice was guided by a profound respect for my patients' autonomy. In the past, doctors felt a moral duty to do what was in the best interests of their patients, even if it meant disregarding their patients' personal inclinations. But the era of the physician's words being gospel has ended, and patients are becoming actively involved in their own care. While a patient enters the therapeutic relationship as the one with less power, physicians can strive to empower their patients to make their own decisions.

Author of the ground-breaking *Anatomy of an Illness*, Norman Cousins believed that "the only answer has to be increased education about the way the human body works, so that more people will be able to steer an intelligent course between promiscuous pill-popping and irresponsible disregard of genuine symptoms" (Cousins, N., 1979, p.101). He was a forceful advocate of his own healthcare plan and eventually found a doctor who would go along with his ideas. While there are patients who need to be directed and wish to be told what to do, I believe that getting a patient to take more responsibility for their healthcare is preferable.

One of my patients who epitomized Norman Cousins' approach of self-directed care was a man who came to me looking for a new diabetologist because his former doctor, a well-recognized expert at a prestigious institution, could not support his diabetic regimen. Granted, this regimen was unique in that he did not want to vary his insulin regimen using short-acting insulin but preferred to use exercise on a trampoline to correct any major blood sugar excursions caused by stress or diet (which was rare because his diet was regimented). He did a good job of monitoring his blood sugar in order to chart his course. I was still seeing this patient when I retired, and he did have some diabetic complications involving his eyes and kidneys, but he had lived with insulin-requiring diabetes for approximately fifty-five years, a tremendous feat. When he first started insulin, the syringes were reused and needed to be sterilized, and sugar was only tested in the urine. The man was to be commended for taking good care of himself under such difficult circumstances, and I had no compunctions about letting him direct his care. Moreover, it was clear that supporting his autonomy was critical to his success. He took pride in living with diabetes for so long and continuing to function so well. And it is uncertain how much his physical health would have been improved by micromanaging his blood sugar control. A holistic approach taking into account his motivations and sense of self would probably benefit him more. There is always some degree of tension between the beneficence of the physician and the autonomy of the patient, but with this patient, it was clear to me that respect for his autonomy was paramount.

Respect for my patients' autonomy did not mean that I kowtowed to all their whims. An interesting situation that illustrates the tension between control and permissiveness has to do with the treatment of anorexics. I helped institute a protocol for severe anorexics in the psych ward at our hospital. In the beginning, it was essential that patients relinquish their control in order to gain much needed weight and draw back from the brink of death. The treatment was by no means a cure. Designing a treatment plan that is effective in the long-term is extremely difficult, and most medical doctors are loath to have anorexics as patients for this reason. My experience, however, was that many of the patients got better over time if given the emotional and psychological support they need in a nonjudgmental way. One of the most dangerously ill of my patients was a woman who weighed 60 pounds when admitted to the hospital and 80 pounds when discharged—not ideal but probably livable. Over the many years I saw her, she was able to maintain her weight in the 90-pound range and become gainfully employed. She felt I was important to her healing from severe physical and emotional abuse and had facilitated her reintegration into society. But I had imposed no ostensible treatments, and there were no appropriate billing codes for what I had done: respect her autonomy and suspend judgment. Mostly, I had tried to be present to her as her journey unfolded.

Sometimes, patients came to me having given over too much of their power to doctors. I then saw it as my job to help them assert a certain measure of independence and take greater control of their health. There was, for example, the case of a young woman who had developed episodes of dread, with difficulty concentrating. She came to see me because her salivary cortisol was low, and her healthcare provider had suggested she might have an adrenal problem. Ironically, it is possible that the adrenal support preparation she'd been given had suppressed her endogenous adrenal output. In any case, my feeling was that she was relying too much on doctors and their medicines to solve her dis-ease. She was able to do hot yoga with no fatigue, and emotionally, she seemed to be coping well with the raising of her two young children. I discussed the insignificance of the salivary cortisol test and proposed she start breathing exercises and meditation as an adjunct to her yoga practice. She resonated well with my suggestions and requested return visits to sharpen her meditation practice, which was of clear benefit to her health and well-being. Again, the problem was how to bill insurance for that!

When is it all right to override the patient's autonomy? Dr. Bernard Lown, a Nobel-Prize-winning physician who wrote *The Lost Art of Healing*, describes an interesting case. He gives an example where he felt it was justified to lie to the patient in order to perform an important electro-conversion. The patient was adamant in her refusal to undergo this potentially life-saving procedure because she was focused on having her back pain addressed first. She did get cardioverted because she was told it would help the back pain even though the doctors did not really believe this.

In general, the doctor must balance attention to the patient's physical health with respect for their personal inclinations and beliefs. To understand these beliefs, communication is essential. A quintessential example of the need for communication is described in the book *The Spirit Catches You and You Fall Down: A Hmong Child, her American Doctors, and the Collision of Two Cultures.* A Hmong child with epilepsy did not take his much-needed epilepsy medication because his parents, following Hmong tradition, understood epilepsy to be the result of possession by spirits. The consequences were fatal. If only there had been more communication and more listening to help bridge the cultural gap.

I was seeing a ninety-year-old Chinese architect who had moved to the US to be close to his son. He was a vibrant man with great intelligence, but he had never learned much English. He came to our visits with his devoted son, who decided that, even though I was seeing his father just for hypothyroidism, I should be his primary physician. When the patient developed prostate cancer, his son and I talked about treatment options. The father was never involved. Normally, I would have made sure that my patient received all the details of a diagnosis and potential treatments and weighed in on any decisions, but in this case, it was clear that the son had complete authority over his father's life, and I chose to respect this cultural difference.

I'm reminded of a movie by Akira Kurosawa called *Ikiru*. It is about a civil servant who goes in for a medical checkup and discovers he has stomach cancer. The physicians are brusque and offer little support. He leaves the clinic knowing he is going to die, but he can tell neither his family nor friends because of the cultural taboo around malignancy. He experiences an epiphany that prompts him to change his life dramatically, and at his funeral, everyone talks about how in his final year, he lived an exemplary life and became an inspiration. They speculate as to the reasons for his personality change, being entirely ignorant of his diagnosis. To me, this film was revelatory in showcasing cultural differences in our attitudes towards disease, what it means and how we treat it.

My visits abroad, as a part of the People-to-People exchange of physicians organized by the State Department, were extremely informative in this regard. During this trip, to Holland, Sweden, Germany, and Russia, I saw first-hand how countries around the world have developed different approaches to medical care as a result of different cultural norms and expectations. Across the world, the body is observed and described in radically different ways. Chinese medicine, for example, distinguishes a much larger variety of head-aches compared to Western medicine, and its descriptive terms of hot and cold have nothing to do with temperature but refer to qi energy instead. Their language, like every language, is a lens through which they see and interpret the world differently. Members of the Blackfeet Nation describe the world using verbs rather than nouns. One can only imagine how their understanding of healing is affected if what they perceive is movement and flow rather than static objects.

If a doctor wishes to promote the healing of a patient from a different culture, it is crucial to take into consideration differences in how they see and describe the world. As a physician, I worked on listening to my patients intently and developing a complete picture of the person before me. If I didn't, I might leap to conclusions, make assumptions, and become a victim to bias. Physicians humble enough to admit their vulnerability can practice the self-awareness necessary to notice and rectify their biases wherever possible. This requires spend-ing enough time with patients, and it means listening carefully with an open mind. Without diligent self-monitoring, without taking the time to observe and then correct first impressions, all the diagnostic acumen in the world will not be enough. If the art of medicine is to be saved, medical training must take into account skills and practices that lie beyond the scientific.

In general, positive outcomes are so much more than a matter of diagnosis and cure. Uncovering the answers to a patient's dis-ease using scientific observation is important, and certainly I had my share of eureka moments, but equally important is the communion and communication. Most visits in a primary care practice don't require probing for esoteric or complicated answers. What is required is the practice of certain virtues—humility and open-mindedness, patience and equanimity, compassion and loving kindness. My highest desire is that these virtues become honored and cherished and understood to be integral to the practice of medicine.

EMR AND AI VERSUS
THE HUMAN PRESENCE

If the art of medicine is to be saved, we must acknowledge the central importance of the patient-doctor relationship and of the psychological aspects of healing. We must acknowledge the profound effects of compassion, humility, patience, and even a sense of humor. We must acknowledge the power of our words in directly affecting our patient's healing. Unfortunately, these qualities get short shrift in a hectic medical world filled with regulations and data overload. The focus is on labeling the disease and assigning a DSM code, but sometimes, the issue is dis-ease, without any constellation of findings leading to a clear diagnosis. In general, the system of electronic medical records leads to a diminished, compartmentalized, fragmented account of the visit in addition to taking away from the visit itself. How can an MD get the data into the system and still gaze into the patient's eyes and offer solace or understanding?

I started practice in the 1970s before the computer age. During my thirty-five years in the field, computer usage soared. The switch to Electronic Medical Records (EMR) was incentivized financially by the Obama administration at the beginning of the Great Recession, partly in order to fuel the recovery. Immediately, multiple issues arose. The system served to maximize medical charges rather than lead to accurate narratives of a visit. In addition, various EMRs were launched without a common platform, so the record could not be universally accessed. Finally, the doctor was supposed to be inputting information while seeing the patient, effectively turning visits into a threesome—doctor, patient, and computer. I personally refused to have the computer in my exam room and instead spent time afterwards doing the inputting required.

The situation has improved with better software and more access and compatibility. And certainly, we no longer have to worry about illegible handwriting, for which some doctors are notorious. But at what cost? A system of endless checkboxes, meant to simplify, leads to mindless inputting. Not only do click fatigue and data input error become a serious problem, but doctors are also prevented from providing more accurate, nuanced records. Often, my colleagues' records would be so disjointed, I could not figure out what had actually occurred during the visit. And as regards my own notes, EMR was so extraordinarily time-consuming and depersonalizing, taking away from my interaction with patients, that it hastened my decision to retire. I'm by no means alone in this. A 2020 study, authored by doctors from the University of Toronto and the Centre for Addiction and Mental Health, found that three-fourths of queried physicians said that electronic health records contributed to their burnout.

Medicine has a strong tradition of storytelling, including a narrative rendition of a healthcare visit. However, the richness and relevance of the story is getting lost as checkboxes and numbers take over. There is no room left for information gleaned from the patient. Dr. Pincus argues that such "subjective" information is vital. It "should not be regarded as supplementary or peripheral to 'objective' physical examinations, radiographs, laboratory tests, and other traditional sources of data concerning patient status, but rather should be seen as an integral, if not an essential component of patient care" (Pincus, 1997, p.25).

What of the role of artificial intelligence? Clearly, it can be an aid in sifting through all the available data. And it can to some extent decrease human error. Artificial intelligence can markedly improve the analysis of mammograms, for example. Studies have shown that radiologists rereading an X-ray contradict themselves almost 20% of the time. Meanwhile, a method called "a random-forest classifier," used at MIT, decreased unnecessary surgeries and increased the diagnosis rate of cancerous lesions from 79 to 97 percent. There are also computer systems using AI that can diagnosis skin disorders better than most dermatologists.

There is, however, a concern that physicians will become dependent on these aids and lose their skills. Also, they may become over-influenced by the computer analysis and fail to consider other possibilities. Certainly, we don't want AI taking the place of human interaction and communication. While at times, artificial intelligence may outperform physicians in physical observation, the highest rates of success occur when doctor and AI work together in a synergistic fashion. Developers are working to improve AI's ability to align to fluid and complex human values and preferences, but even so, we cannot allow it to make the final decision. It can be used as an aid but not as the final arbiter. Ideally, it will give physicians more time to relate to patients.

Science will continue to advance, and technology will continue to develop new ways for us to manage our practice, but the cornerstone of medical care will always be its humanity. Nothing can substitute for the doctor as a human presence. A revealing study provided anesthesiologists with two scripts. Both communicated what the patient needed to know before undergoing surgery, but one was more personal and interactive. The more socially interactive group left the hospital a day and a half earlier and required less pain medicine (Egbert, L.D.,1964). Clearly, the briefest of human connections can have a tremendous effect.

At a Washington State Medical conference, a short play was performed to communicate the importance of heartfelt human interaction. It described how traditional medical school training, by concentrating solely on the analysis of facts, creates doctors who display neither the desire nor the skill to interact with their patients in a meaningful way. Maureen Manley acted her own story while another actor played the part of the doctor. At the age of twenty-six, Maureen was a world-class bicyclist. During the Women's Tour De France, she developed some blurriness of vision and, becoming imbalanced, fell off her bike. She tried to continue but could not. Devastated, she returned to the United States to find out what was wrong. She was given the diagnosis of multiple sclerosis, which is not always easy to determine. She had already seen several doctors when a young neurologist gave her the bad news. The play describes the doctor's story in addition to hers, showing him making his way through medical school before his fateful encounter with Maureen. When he first entered medical school, he was idealistic, with a strong humanistic and poetic nature, but after going through the medical fact factory, with its rigorous, austere interactions, he became an intelligent, dispassionate physician.

The final scene in his office shows him telling Maureen that her diagnosis is multiple sclerosis and that she should come back to discuss the treatment plan. Having presented her with the data, he walks out of the room. Maureen is left alone, distraught, and bewildered as the lights go out. The truth is, she was alone even in his presence. The doctor was no more human than a system of artificial intelligence would have been.

The play clearly demonstrates a fundamental deficit of our system of medical education, in particular the absence of humanity. At the University of Washington, I became part of the Healer's Art Program, developed by the psychiatrist Rachel Naomi Remen to address this deficiency. A remarkable woman who had had much of her intestine surgically removed due to Crohn's Disease, she promoted the integration of the mind, body, and soul for optimal medical care and coined the term Wounded Healer. Her writing includes the best seller *Kitchen Table Wisdom*, a collection of narratives of dying patients that emphasizes the need for resolution with family members before passing. This book is heartfelt, as was her course. A small group of medical students attended, and they were divided into groups, with about five students per facilitator. The idea was to create an intimate environment for the sharing of grief, loss, and other emotions. If students could get in touch with their own experiences, they would be more comfortable and compassionate when hearing patients discuss their problems. Understanding feelings and attitudes was the goal of our meetings, with topics such as selfcare; relationships that support selfcare; relationships that are nonjudgmental, noncompetitive, and collegial; and the power of listening. Meetings bore such titles as "Mystery and Awe" and "Care of the Soul." The exposure of students to material that was non-scientific and non-factual was a critical addition to the general medical curriculum. It was a direct attempt to teach the art of medicine.

THE TEAM AND COMMUNITY

I have been discussing the one-on-one relationship of doctors with their patients, but no doctor works in a vacuum. Practicing the art of medicine requires the support of a team as well as the cultivation of relationships within the greater community.

At my office, the attitude of my staff was essential to the delivery of high-quality healthcare. From the receptionists making appointments and greeting the patients, to the personnel in charge of the charts, everyone worked together in a friendly, compassionate, supportive atmosphere, pervaded by mutual respect and care for the patient. We were like a family, enjoying birthday celebrations at the office and Halloween and other holiday events at the physicians' homes.

My success absolutely depended on the caring and knowledgeable clinical staff that surrounded me. That said, my medical assistant was the one who was most critical. Over a period of fourteen years, I had six medical assistants, and then Patty was hired as a new graduate. Over a twenty-year period, she became a proficient provider of health-care with a knowledge base that exceeded that of many a diabetic nurse practitioner, and she was a caring soul devoted to the welfare of our patients. Normally, medical assistants would simply be responsible for rooming patients, but not in this case. She was involved in every aspect of care, from downloading and collecting blood sugars recorded by meters or CGM devices to starting patients on insulin or other home injectables; from answering questions regarding diabetic care, on the phone or in person to triaging and determining urgency of care. Patty developed close relationships with many of our patients and even when they moved out of state, they stayed in touch for personal reasons or to ask for clinical advice, in consultation with me, of course. She and I worked together like dance partners, each of us knowing what the next step would be.

The other healthcare provider with whom I developed a special relationship was Emily, a diabetic nurse practitioner who had Type 1. It would not be possible to have a colleague with more knowledge and practical wisdom. She understood diabetic management from every angle, personally and practically. We undertook several projects together to enrich the lives of the diabetic patient. Sponsored by the Kent Lions Club, we developed a manual for pregnancy planning for women with diabetes. Emily was well-equipped to spearhead this undertaking since she had been an early user of the insulin pump during her two pregnancies. She emphasized the need to be well-prepared with good blood sugar control before getting pregnant to avoid playing catch up.

I was a member of other amazing teams. Some healthcare problems by their very nature require a broader base of healthcare support. One early, highly coordinated team effort in which I participated was the inpatient treatment of anorexia, a program I discussed earlier. These patients had severe control issues and were in dire physical straits, emaciated as well as malnourished. The immediate goal was improving caloric intake for survival. They would be admitted to the psych unit with a staff of psych aides, nurses, and psychiatrists. I was the medical director and oversaw the protocol for refeeding and monitoring caloric intake, with significant involvement by dietitians and a pharmacist. Sometimes, invasive nutrition treatments were needed, requiring NG tube feeding or in extreme cases, central IV placement for total parental nutrition. The patients had to give up their autonomy and accept the protocol, but they could be very manipulative, so it was all the more important for the staff to remain cohesive and focused on our goals. Also, the patients were constantly flirting with death, willing to harm themselves in order to perversely maintain control. Needless to say, this caused the staff tremendous stress. It took tremendous team effort for everyone to get through.

Teams are essential to healthcare in another way as well. Support groups of various kinds with different modes of operation are recognized as essential to healing, including AA, Al-Anon, and a multitude of groups for specific ailments. Emily and I were personally involved in the development of the Washington State Teenage Diabetic Support System, under the auspices of the Washington State chapter of the American Diabetic Association. Our model was to pair a well-adjusted, diabetic teenager with other diabetic teenagers who were struggling to take care of themselves. We worked with high school counselors to identify both the kids that needed support and those who could serve as supportive friends. Every year, we would organize a day-long retreat to offer the "together" teenagers, teachings on how to encourage their struggling peers without judging their behaviors. Facilitators trained in psychology would lead bonding exercises to make the experience fun rather than didactic. The advice was to make friends with the diabetic compatriot while letting go of the need to give specific advice on the "correct" way of doing treatment. Eventually, the Washington State ADA took over the program completely, and there were some feelers from other chapters of the ADA for further implementation.

Another program in which I participated also stressed the importance of support. I was the medical director of one of the sites of the Health Management Resources liquid diet program. (In the 1990s, quick weight loss in a highly regulated system was in vogue, the other major organization being Optifast.) In groups of about ten patients, a liquid diet of 600 calories was instituted, with frequent laboratory testing and an intensive, educational program focused on exercise and calorie-counting. Facilitators from the diet and exercise physiology fields promoted bonding via weekly meetings to maximize short-term and (hopefully) long-term weight loss. Participants lost from 50 to 250 pounds before a gradual refeeding program was started, six to nine months after the initiation of the liquid diet. The idea was that quick weight loss would be very gratifying for the subjects and help them develop the confidence that would lead to long-term success. Unfortunately, even though many participants were in refeeding for a whole year and intensely supported by the staff and other patients, many regained over half their weight back. The program had quick results, but only small to moderate rewards in the long term. I mention this to show that while team and community efforts are essential, they are not the whole picture.

One of the first studies examining the importance of group support was performed in the late 1980s by Dr. Spiegel, involving metastatic breast cancer patients. The follow-up was over a ten-year period after patients had received a year of weekly support group sessions, led by a psychiatrist or social worker and a therapist who had breast cancer in remission. Only three patients were alive at the end of the observation period, but survival had doubled: 36 months with psychosocial support compared to 18 months with the control group. The clinical trial made clear what so many of us already know: the importance of companionship and camaraderie in bolstering good health.

A fascinating study of two communities in Pennsylvania similarly suggests that people's health is profoundly affected by their experience of connectedness. It showed that during the period 1955–1965, the town of Roseto in Pennsylvania had a dramatically lower mortality rate for heart attacks compared to surrounding towns. Known risk factors for cardiovascular disease, such as diet, smoking, and occupation, were similar in nearby towns, but what distinguished Roseto was its close-knit, Italian culture—the town had been settled in 1882 by immigrants from southern Italy. It appeared that a cohesive family unit led to better cardiovascular outcomes. This result was supported by a subsequent study showing that from 1965 to 1974, a period during which social cohesion had weakened significantly, the health benefit disappeared.

The *National Geographic* "Blue Zones" project, spanning a decade and a half, identified five "hotspots of longevity," which had an unusual number of centenarians, and was able to connect their good health with social contact. Admittedly, other factors could explain the findings, including genetics, exercise, and diet, two of the hotspots being in the region where the Mediterranean diet is consumed, for instance. Loma Linda, California, with the highest concentration of Seventh Day Adventists in the US, and Nicoya Peninsula, Costa Rica, with strong faith communities, were clearly distinguished by their strong, social networks. The fifth spot, Okinawa, Japan, had a unique system of social support groups known as *moais*. Infants from different families form bonds as if they were siblings, embedding families in an extended meshwork of caring and companionship.

Social cohesion should be on the list of health activities, right up with exercycles and kale smoothies. In the United States, unfortunately, loneliness is an epidemic, one that started long before the coronavirus pandemic. We would do well to learn from the Danes and the value they give to "hygge," something that is hard to define but has to do with both coziness and togetherness and engenders a profound feeling of contentedness. Perhaps it contributes to Denmark's being ranked, at various times, the happiest country on earth.

A doctor can have a great rapport with their patients, but without outside support and assistance, a doctor's efforts may be insufficient, even futile. I've mentioned my encounters during medical school with Latina teenagers who were deprived of almost all social contacts and became psychotic. As practitioners of medicine, we must acknowledge the effect of community on the health of our patients and do all we can to connect our patients with communities of support.

CHAPTER SEVEN

Therapeutic Interventional Potential—Mind Over Matter

Growing up, I embraced the scientific paradigm, and yet I found the answers it provided to be incomplete and sterile. There was no role for the individual psyche. There was no discussion of the one who is interpreting the universe and that person's subjectivity. This realm fascinated me from the beginning. As a kid in high school, I was enamored with Freud and read most of his works about the id, ego, and superego and how the dynamics among these, shape our understanding of reality. I was also an avid reader of D.H. Lawrence. This was back in the '60s when the sexual revolution was beginning to unfold. As a teenage boy, I was titillated by the subject of sexuality, but more importantly, there was a passion in Lawrence's writings that I could not find in the studious, erudite presentation of cases by Freud. They both talked about sexual desire, but to me, Lawrence was more alive and in touch with life itself.

Lawrence himself drew attention to their differences, presenting in a book called *The Fantasia of the Unconscious* his thoughts and feelings about Freudian psychology. He ranted about how its rational, mind-based approach ignored our humanity. Lawrence came up with his own convoluted system in which the solar plexus is the hub of understanding, not the mind. Despite the impassioned, vituperative statements about Freudian dogma, Lawrence's approach was a holistic one that I found refreshing. "It is life we have to live by, not machines and ideals. And life means nothing else, even, but the spontaneous living soul which is our central reality. The spontaneous, living, individual soul… All the rest is derived" (Lawrence, 1960, p.183).

SYSTEMS OF BELIEF

Understanding the whole as a sacrosanct entity that cannot be constructed by assembling its parts has always seemed to me essential in tackling any problem. And certainly, in medicine, this is true. Materialism—"what you see is what you get"—is wholly inadequate as a belief system, and yet, it is the easiest to adopt. People are quick to accept the primacy of objects and respect the information and conclusions gleaned using our physical senses. Science in isolation is a reductionistic system that focuses on the pieces to fit them into a bigger picture. In medicine, this means that the body is fragmented and our understanding of how the body works and how it may be healed is needlessly restricted.

In my view, science is as much a belief system as any philosophical system. Its ideal is objectivity, and subjectivity is to be eradicated. But it is commonplace knowledge that our culture and upbringing shape our reality. And physics itself teaches us that the observer changes what is observed. Heisenberg's uncertainty principle suggests that reality is defined by the dyad of object and observer. Knowledge becomes a dance. In the realm of medicine, this means that the patient-doctor relationship cannot be ignored—reality itself is shaped by this relationship.

There is a parable that beautifully describes the two distinct approaches:

Two men of different persuasions, Ari and Zen, are walking down a path with Ari having complete command of Aristotelian logic and scientific methodology while Zen is a contemplative master. Along the path, they encounter two identical flowers that they wish to understand. With tremendous relish and energy, Ari applies himself to the task. He picks the flower in order to conduct innumerable analytic tests, gathering all the particular information possible regarding "What is this flower?" It is an exhaustive enterprise leading to a vast accumulation of complex data filling multiple volumes. Ari feels satisfied that the flower is now totally appreciated and walks on, while the object of study no longer exists, except in a tome of particulars and details. (Perhaps he presses the remnants between the pages of his notebook.)

Zen approaches the remaining flower and sits down, gazing at it. He spends a considerable amount of time contemplating it, using both his physical senses and an intuitive awareness of his connection to the flower. He observes the environment in which the flower grows as well as other contexts—of history and meaning. There is a deep rapport between himself and the flower. After an indeterminate amount of time, Zen gets up, satisfied that the flower is now known. That second flower remains after Zen's departure. The question is "Who knows the flower?"

Of course, there is no correct answer, and both sides can claim to have the better perspective. Obliterating the flower to understand it might well feel antithetical to its ultimate meaning; at the same time, having a purely personal experience without gleaning any objective information and seeing the flower as inseparable from its context might be considered a very inadequate result.

Another interesting question is: Is there any part of Zen's experience that cannot be found in Ari's data base? Can a computer containing all the gathered information "know" the flower the way Zen does? The word "qualia" represents the part that is left out, the subjective conscious experience, which is ineffable, private, and cannot be accessed by science but only by the individual. The classic example of "qualia" is the quality of redness. If someone knew everything about redness—its wavelength, etc.—but had never had the experience of seeing anything red, he/she could hardly appreciate what "red" is.

The scientific method zeroes in on the parts, which undergo rigorous examination and are then put together to construct an edifice of knowledge that is polished and shimmers with correctitude. The universe, it seems, does not exist outside of this edifice. With a more spiritual approach, which does not have to be religious and include a god or creator, the universe is present from the beginning, and we are discoverers within it. In 1972, James Lovelock, a futurist, proposed the Gaia hypothesis, which holds that organic and inorganic entities are all connected in a synergistic, unified structure as basically one life form. Again, one does not have to be religious to understand the universe in this way, although it does seem to be the belief underlying all religions that there is a unity from which all is created, and thus, deep down, we are all connected.

For millennia, it was spirituality and not science that was considered the ultimate path of understanding. The spirit is that which lies beyond material existence and the ken of the five senses. Science would seem to be the antithesis of spirituality, but great scientists have often spoken with awe and reverence of a holistic universe that an approach like Ari's cannot capture. Einstein argued for a broader understanding. When a rabbi wrote him in 1950 that he'd sought in vain to comfort his daughter over the death of her younger sister, Einstein replied that "a human being is part of the whole, called by us 'Universe'… He experiences himself, his thoughts and feelings as something separate from the rest—a kind of optical delusion of his consciousness. This delusion is a kind of a prison for us, restricting us to our personal desires and to affection for a few persons nearest us. Our task must be to free ourselves from this prison by widening our circle of compassion to embrace all living creatures and the whole of nature in its beauty."

While some scientists aim for absolute knowledge, with physicists such as Sean Carroll believing that the laws of the physical universe can be completely known, others like David Bohm espouse what I consider a more spiritual view. A theoretical physicist with access to the same information as Carroll, he suggested that there exists an infinite potential from which everything else is generated. Offering no starting point in time and space, the concept is abstract and, since it can be neither proven nor disproven, appears irrelevant in the world of scientific justification. Then again, scientific dogma has not been able to reconcile the theory of relativity, which describes the macro-universe, with the theory of quantum mechanics, which describes the micro-universe. So, clearly there is much that lacks explanation.

Science and spirituality need not be antithetical. Bohm himself had an intimate connection with Krishnamurti, an Indian philosopher who was probing the nature of mind using meditation, holistic inquiry, and an understanding of human relationships, and their conversations were published in *The Ending of Time: Where Philosophy and Physics Meet*. The Dalai Lama frequently expresses his respect for science and has been integral in building bridges of mutual enquiry and understanding between the two camps. His Mind and Life Symposia have brought together preeminent scientists and spiritual practitioners.

Bohm's words are worth repeating: "Whatever we say anything is, it isn't." As soon as we think we know reality, it exceeds us. With this as an underlying credo, one becomes more open to alternative avenues of exploration. As just one example, there is the phenomenon of synchronicity that you yourself have perhaps experienced. There are many stories of loved ones dying or in danger while someone else, without being present, is nonetheless aware of it.

I have had the experience of someone I had not been thinking about for a year call me right after I mentioned that person to someone else. Similarly, once I went to a movie with a fellow medical resident, and we jested about having never experienced an usher yelling, "Is there a doctor in the house?" Right after our conversation, that is exactly what happened. Do we assume such events are pure coincidence, or can we be open to something else going on? What if the world is not the purely materialistic universe we assume it is?

Einstein is often quoted as saying that "the world we have created is a product of our thinking; it cannot be changed without changing our thinking. If we want to change the world we have to change our thinking... We must learn to see the world anew." Such dramatic changes in perception are paradigm shifts; they feel revelatory. From another perspective, they are symptoms of our thinking having become incapacious, of how we've confined ourselves to a set of beliefs so rigid that it can only be changed by a rupture that is sudden and dramatic.

An alternative is to always see the truth as provisional rather than absolute. It means that we never really know if anything is true. This is the attitude that I personally subscribe to. Richard Feynman writes, "I can live with doubt and uncertainty and not knowing. I think it is much more interesting to live not knowing than to have answers that might be wrong. If we will only allow that, as we progress, we remain unsure, we will leave opportunities for alternatives." I prefer, as Feynman does, to "keep the door to the unknown ajar" (Feynman, 2010).

My medical journey has been one of refining my science but at same time connecting to a deep humility regarding the limitations of my knowledge. Letting go of the illusion of objectivity, I found myself on paths that took me beyond science and its focus on facts. I cultivated other attitudes and capabilities, transforming my ideas around what constitutes healthcare. Medical practice involves the practice of so much else besides good science. If we can open to the breadth of what is possible, our health and well-being will be profoundly improved.

MEDITATION

In the fall of 1992, something happened that would alter my course dramatically. Robert Frost in his poem "The Road Not Taken" said it best.

> Two roads diverged in a wood, and I—
> I took the one less traveled by,
> And that has made all the difference.

I had finished cleaning leaves off the roof of our house and was lowering myself onto the ladder when I accidentally kicked it away. My fall would only have been nine feet, but I grabbed the corrugated gutter. That night, the hand surgeon told me I had severed eight tendons. He could try to repair the injured right hand by making the tendons either lax for full extension of my fingers or tight for a strong grip. He was basically asking me whether I wanted to continue playing piano or tennis. I chose tennis.

Three surgeries were performed over eighteen months to correct contractures. When locked in a special contraption, my fingers stayed extended, but they promptly lost extension during rehab. Perhaps, I was not as good a patient as I could have been to prevent the contractures from recurring. Anyway, with two of my favorite activities no longer available, I became open to other possibilities and embarked on a completely new path. I joined a men's group reading Robert Bly and started a meditation practice.

I decided to share my newly established meditation practices with my patients as a focusing and relaxing exercise. I quickly realized, however, how impractical it was to teach meditation during an office visit. Physicians were under pressure at the time to cut medical visits to seven minutes to improve efficiency. This confluence of circumstances led to a eureka moment. I needed to focus on my personal practice rather than pushing it on my patients. A strong meditation practice would help me to become more attentive and present. The quality of our interaction would improve, and ultimately, I would accomplish more in a shorter amount of time.

It took time for me to develop my meditation practice, which was steeped in Buddhist teachings and not simply mindfulness. Buddhism is not a religion so much as a philosophy of the mind, a path to deeper understanding of the human condition and human consciousness. There are also tenets for living and acting from an ethical point of view. I was never a zealot and had no desire to proselytize. I simply wanted to embody my practice as fully as I could, bringing to my interaction with others a spiritual quality having to do with the unity and connection of all human beings. The outcome was more compassion, caring, and love. I also undertook a group of meditation practices, which helped focus the mind. I soon realized that these practices enhanced my ability to observe and analyze a patient's condition. Also enhanced was my ability to observe myself and my emotions, allowing me to handle interpersonal relationships more judiciously and compassionately.

Buddhist principles can be incorporated into a philosophy of life independent of any formal religious practice. For me, the aim was to meld the scientific with the spiritual, medical expertise with harmony and love. In 2005, I attended a Mind and Life Conference on "The Science and Clinical Applications of Meditation." It was a revelation to me on how Buddhist thought can work successfully with science to explore the workings of the mind. Jon Kabat-Zinn discussed his work with Mindfulness-Based Stress Reduction (MBSR), a meditation practice that does not require formal Buddhist training. In MBSR as well as Mindfulness-Based Cognitive Therapy (MBCT) developed by Segal, Williams, and Teasdale, subjects pay close attention to their thoughts, moods, sensations, and emotions without judgment; they are present to what is unfolding in each and every moment. Mindfulness has become a household word. And over time, thousands of studies have demonstrated its positive impact on people's well-being, mental as well as physical, including the immune system and cardiac functioning, among others.

At the conference, Richie Davidson, a professor of psychology as well as director of the Laboratory for Affective Neuroscience at University of Wisconsin, presented a study comparing three groups: long-term meditators, new meditators who had taken an eight-week MBSR course, and a control group who had taken a course in well-being practices with no mention of meditation. They were asked to view and label photos as either emotionally positive, negative, or neutral. As measured by MRIs, both the new and long-term meditators demonstrated less emotional reactivity to positive images, but only the seasoned meditators had decreased reactivity to negative images.

I began to dream of the general medical community incorporating meditation practices into its health plans. Unfortunately, Western medicine has never fully appreciated the power of the mind in affecting physical health. There has only been some lip service in that direction. Other cultures show a more profound understanding. During my visit to China, I was struck by the number of people in the park practicing Tai Chi—several hundred. They clearly understood the connection between mind and body.

In order to learn more about Buddhism, I visited Dharamsala, India, the seat of the Tibetan state in exile, and took part in a three-day teaching with the Dalai Lama. Meditation is an individual grounding that is enhanced in a group setting, and I have been involved in various sanghas—communities of like-minded individuals who engage in Buddhist practices together—throughout my twenty-five years of meditation practice. The one most relevant here is the Healthcare Meditation Group, inspired by the Dalai Lama's "Seeds of Compassion" visit to Seattle in 2008. Healthcare providers meet once a month to meditate, offer mutual support, and explore topics having to do, not with the science of medicine, but with the care of ourselves and our patients.

For many years, I was the chief facilitator of the group. For one of the exercises, I requested that the members write down their thoughts regarding the impact of their meditation practice on their practice of healthcare. The next meeting, these comments were collated anonymously and handed out to the group for discussion. They reveal fascinating interconnections between the two practices. Here is a sampling:

Meditation has allowed me to listen deeply to patients and detach myself from personal thoughts and worries. I am a lot more present with my patients and can suspend my judgments and just BE there compassionately. This compassion is also for me. I try to do the best I can for others, but the patient is not always appreciative of my efforts. A letter from a disgruntled patient accused me of not addressing her problem. I looked over my notes, showing that I had tried to give her a perspective on her problems. This patient will probably not come back, but I hope that she does so we can further explore her needs. Meditation helps me to reconsider the patient's view in a new light. If the patient was discontented and felt she did not receive the help she needed, then more exploration was needed to alleviate her suffering. Negative emotions suggest a need for further investigation and do not indicate failure.

I like to use my meditation practice to calm myself when in the presence of agitated or angry people. I focus on my breathing and deliberately slow it down. This helps me to remain calm and present and to listen more deeply. It has helped me both professionally and in my personal life. When I remain fully present, I am not thinking about me. I am totally focused on the patient, and they sense this. It helps them to eventually calm down as well and to speak their truth.

What is meditation: a way to shed the "buzz" of life, to connect with what is fundamental. How to use it: for patients in mid-workup to help them concentrate on what they can control, to stay with the present moment and not worry about the "what ifs." Also, when patients are dissatisfied or upset and venting/ranting, I remind myself to breathe and remember that I can show care instead of being reactive.

Meditation strengthens my ability to be totally present in each encounter, more in touch, to have compassion for the distress and suffering of the patient. It clarifies my clinical judgment, strengthens my cognition and ability to learn, integrate, and use new information, allows me to be much more mindful in many areas, including how much time I am spending with the patient and how the patient is reacting. In the past year, I have sensed much more connection with my patients, and so many of them seem truly touched and grateful for the services.

Meditation is a way to cultivate Awareness and Presence, knowing who we are in essence, feeling the preciousness of this life, no matter what hardships or conflicts arise physically, emotionally, mentally, or spiritually. I can bring meditation into healing by resonating that sense of wholeness with others so that they too can feel and get in touch with their wholeness. It's a way of offering people the space and confidence to experience who they are beyond the pain of our human condition.

I have found that meditation and mindfulness allow me to stay present and focused on each patient without any distraction or thought as to what has occurred previously or what is awaiting me after this meeting. I believe that when we are providing care to patients, we are conduits of healing.

What I do to be a better practitioner, friend, mom is to empty—to be spacious so as not to let the worrisome and fearful thoughts invade and take over and to help those who suffer to become more spacious and live in the present moment, so that fear has less of a grip on us all.

Because we're healthcare providers, people share their suffering with us. Our meditation practice helps us to take it in and help them. Without a foundation in meditation, we are more like a sponge that is still in its cellophane wrap—we can't really take in the suffering and are not able to help much.

Several years after retiring, I visited the Rainier Clinical Research Center I had founded decades earlier. Imagine my surprise and delight when I saw in the entryway a Zen garden.

BELIEFS, ATTITUDES, AND PLACEBOS

As I developed my spiritual practice, I became increasingly aware of mind-body medicine and the extraordinary amount of work conducted by the scientific community to understand and describe this connection. A study of London taxicab drivers, for example, revealed that learning to navigate a complex grid of streets had physically changed their brains—MRIs showed that the hippocampal areas involved with spatial memory were enlarged. The idea of exercising to get stronger and more skilled physically is recognized by everyone, but meditation also influences emotional intelligence, awareness, alertness, and well-being, in ways that are often physically manifest. There are numerous studies regarding the effects of mind training on depression, chronic pain, and anxiety. The studies are often small, and criticisms of biases are leveled by skeptical reviewers, but, as we have seen, the supposedly objective RCTs are just as vulnerable to bias.

Psychoneuroimmunology (and endocrinology can be included here) is the scientific field that attempts to understand the body in a more holistic way, investigating the interplay of mind, hormones, the immune system, and the environment, internal as well as external. It is a difficult realm to study in the traditional manner since the object of study—the mind—is not detectable through any of our five senses. No single study makes an incontrovertible case, and the underlying causes and mechanisms remain cloaked in mystery.

Still, a growing number of studies elucidate the connection between the psyche and the immune system. For example, repressed emotions have been associated with a much higher risk of breast cancer. Type A personalities have a much higher incidence of cardiovascular disease. Along the same lines, an examination of Swedish national registry data for 136,637 patients with stress-related disorders revealed that they had a 64% increased incidence of cardiovascular disease compared to match siblings with no mental health diagnosis (Song, H.et al, 2019, p.1255). In Japan, they have ascribed the term *karoshi* to the phenomenon of young workers dying from heart disease or stroke because of the stress of overwork. And I have discussed the physical impacts of social isolation.

A frightening example of the power of thought involves the well-known case of Sam Shoeman, who was diagnosed with esophageal cancer after surgery. A subsequent liver scan revealed extensive metastases, and he was told that he was terminal. Sam wanted to survive past Christmas to be with his relatives and then died right after New Year's Eve. The most remarkable part of the story was that an autopsy showed the scan to have been botched—there was only a small, two-centimeter cancerous nodule, not enough to cause death. It was his belief, and that of everyone around him, that caused his demise (Meador, C. K., 1992, pp.244-247). Many cases of "voodoo" death have been documented, where people, when told they have been cursed, succumb to the death that they believe inevitable.

On the plus side, there are numerous studies that show the potential benefits of belief. In a small study of seventy-six participants, Leibowitz demonstrated that assurances from a healthcare provider mitigated symptoms. Participants were given a histamine skin prick and divided into two groups. The "assurance" group was told, "From this point forward your allergic reaction will start to diminish, and your rash and irritation will go away" (Leibowitz, 2018, p.2051). That simple statement led to a significant decrease in itching compared to the placebo group. The value of positive psychology, first propounded by Dr. Seligman, is clear.

Dr. Becca Levy has spent her academic life studying how psychosocial factors influence cognitive as well as physical functioning. In one fascinating study, elderly patients were exposed to two types of language, associating aging either with wisdom or decline. Words were flashed subliminally: *wise, alert, accomplished, insightful, astute,* etc. for one group and *decline, dependent, dementia, confused, decrepit* for the other. The effect on their performance in subsequent cognitive tests was significant (Levy, 1996, pp.1092-1107). Clearly, a kind word or thought makes a difference, even without conscious processing. While aging is a fact of life, and a good diet and exercise routine can increase longevity, attitude plays an important role. "Age is an issue of mind over matter. If you don't mind, it doesn't matter," Mark Twain is said to have quipped. The implications for a doctor's interaction with his patient—the attitudes conveyed, and the language used—are clearly profound. As a doctor, I always took care to choose my words carefully, knowing their power to affect my patients' beliefs and therefore their health. And I injected humor and lightheartedness wherever possible.

Actively engaging the mind to control the body has great potential in the realm of pain management. These days, limiting the use of opioids is a priority. In a study on pain management in a burn unit, Frank Lawlis revealed the value of relaxation techniques in decreasing pain, with added benefits when imagery was included (Achterberg,1988, p.71). Modern technology can now supercharge imagery by creating completely immersive virtual realities. A burn unit in Seattle, Washington used virtual reality (VR) to control pain with remarkable success. The VR environment was nicknamed SnowWorld because patients felt they were immersed in a snow canyon, with all sounds from the outside world blocked out. Pain was reduced by about half, similar to what an opioid would achieve. (Marchant J., 2014, p.95). These are definitely exciting times as we build up a therapeutic armamentarium that is non-pharmacological and utilizes the natural healing abilities of our body and mind.

The power of the mind to affect the body is well-known in the case of placebos. There is, however, a great deal of paranoia about the placebo effect. Pharmaceutical companies try to minimize or even eliminate this effect in scientifically controlled trials, believing that the efficacy of a medication or procedure cannot otherwise be demonstrated. It is true that, within the context of an RCT, clear conclusions can be muddied by the confounding influence of extra factors. In general, however, the placebo effect is an extraordinary phenomenon that should be exploited for its healing potential.

Throughout the history of pharmacopeia, numerous medicinal products have been shown to have no direct physiologic effect, and yet patients have had a therapeutic response. The Materia Medica is full of half-truths because the benefit of a given medicine was clearly observed even though the reason could have been the psychosocial dynamic between the patient and the healthcare provider. Shamanism, for example, derives much of its success from the extraordinary dynamic between patient and healer as well as the power of a highly choreographed ritual. When there are good results, why should one argue?

Unfortunately, in many parts of the world today, our understanding of the workings of the body has become mostly scientific, and physicians are revered, not for their supernatural powers, but for their scientific acumen. Still, even Western scientists have come to recognize the power of the placebo. In 1955, Henry Beecher wrote in *The Powerful Placebo* that placebos could cause objective changes that even exceed those attributable to potent pharmacologic action. In 1975, Robert Ader demonstrated that after mice received saccharin-flavored water to lessen nausea, alongside an immunosuppressant drug cyclophosphamide, afterwards, the sweetened water alone was able to suppress the white cell count, to the point of mortality. A purely mental association ended up having a lethal effect (Ader, R. & Cohen, N., 1975).

This classic conditioning paradigm works with humans as well. In the 1980s, a young woman with severe lupus was given cyclophosphamide to suppress an overactive immune system that was causing systemic damage to her body, but the medication had such severe side effects that the physicians were willing to try a classic conditioning trial to lower her dosage. Robert Ader and Karen Olness suggested that the medicine be paired with cod liver oil and a rose perfume, two substances with very distinctive sensations. Over the course of a year, she was able to use about half the amount of the drug to get adequate immunosuppression, and eventually she was taken off the drug altogether and put on a less toxic medication. She also stopped the cod liver oil, but she continued to imagine the fragrance of a rose (Olness, K. & Ader, R., 1992).

An early study that demonstrates the power of the placebo was performed by Luparello in 1970. There were four arms to the study, and each participant went through the full protocol, selected randomly. Group 1 received a bronchodilator and Group 3 received a bronchoconstrictor; these have opposite effects, and both groups were correctly informed of the agent they were receiving. Groups 2 and 4, however, were told that they were receiving the opposite of what they were actually given. The results are astounding, for the latter two groups had attenuated responses, approximately half of what was expected. And in some cases, they had no response at all or even the opposite of what the agent would provoke, simply because that was what they believed was going to happen (Luparello et al., 1970). The lesson is that by interjecting negative thoughts in clinical care, a doctor can negate the effects of treatment and even lead to a nocebo effect—a detrimental outcome.

Another researcher, Kaptchuk, designed a study for irritable bowel syndrome in which the subjects were told that they were being given a placebo with the other arm of the study being given nothing at all besides usual care. The placebo was presented in positive terms as a potentially powerful agent with demonstrable effects in various studies, though it was not a medication. The subjects were also told that a positive attitude during the study and taking the placebo pills faithfully would be beneficial. During the three-week randomized trial, symptom severity and relief were statistically improved with the known placebo (Kaptchuk et al, 2010).

An old case study from 1957 that has always intrigued me is the story of Mr. Wright who was diagnosed with lymphoma and had extensive tumor growth throughout his body. Treatments had been ineffectual, and Mr. Wright was open to any new avenue of treatment. Krebiozen was privately made, supposedly from the blood of Argentinean horses injected with a bacterium. His physician reluctantly gave him a shot, and Mr. Wright had a miraculous reaction with all his tumors disappearing. Two months later, the National Cancer Institute reviewed all known Krebiozen-injected patients and concluded no efficacy. When Mr. Wright received this news, his cancer reappeared. His physician was impressed with Mr. Wright's initially positive response and reinjected him with a supposedly highly potent dose of Krebiozen that was, in reality, a water placebo. The tumors responded positively again, but the American Medical Association kept disseminating negative information, and Mr. Wright no longer had the same expectations. The cancer reappeared again, and he succumbed. There are different theories as to what caused the variable course of his disease, but according to psychoneuroimmunologists, lymphomas, compared to other cancers, are more likely to be affected by the mind and expectations (Niemi, 2009).

The power of expectation is elegantly displayed in a study by Burstein on migraines. Half the patients received Maxalt, a well-known migraine medication, and the other half received a placebo. Within these two groups, a third was told they were given a placebo, a third Maxalt or placebo, and the remaining third Maxalt. In the end, receiving the drug (but thinking it was a placebo) and receiving a placebo (but thinking it was the drug) made no difference. There was no difference in pain score if the pill was labeled Maxalt/placebo or Maxalt (Kam-Hansen et al, 2014). Apparently, as long as subjects saw the name of a known active agent and went through the ritual of taking a pill, they gained the benefit—they harbored some expectation of relief.

Studies have been conducted exploring the placebo effect in the realm of mental health as well. It is estimated that up to 75% of the therapeutic effect of antidepressants can be mediated by the placebo response. The psychiatrist's belief in the drug while prescribing it also significantly improves its effect. It appears that the placebo effect enhances the benefit of, not just pharmacological agents, but also psychotherapy. According to Messer and Wampold, who reviewed a wealth of studies as well as meta-analyses, successful therapy is more dependent on certain common factors such as a good therapist-client alliance and the strength of a therapist's belief in their therapy (their allegiance to it) than on the specific type of therapy utilized. This phenomenon is referred to as the "Dodo bird verdict," named after the Dodo in *Alice in Wonderland* who issued a competition and then declared everyone the winner (Luborsky et al., 2002, p.2). A study by Strupp and Hadley compared "therapists" who were well-trained psychotherapists with professors who were renowned for their warmth and trustworthiness. Both groups of clients improved, with no statistical difference between the two (Strupp & Hadley, 1979, p.1125). What was significant was the good therapist-client alliance they had in common. Other studies may have different results, but at the very least, we get a sense of how valuable a kind and thoughtful presence is, within the ritualized context of patient and healer. If doctors are to step fully into their role, clearly, they must accept the psychological aspects of their work.

You may be surprised to learn that even surgery is influenced by the placebo effect. The impressive display of technical expertise has a powerful psychological impact. In the 1950s, internal mammary ligation surgery was performed to increase blood flow to cardiac patients with angina, and it appeared to work. However, a study with a sham operation where an incision of the chest was performed, but no artery was ligated, demonstrated equal efficacy in decreasing anginal pain.

Similar studies have been performed with knee and back surgeries. The grander and more complex the surgery, the greater the placebo effect. Shots have a greater perceived potency than pills. And even the color of pills can magnify the placebo effect.

While the pharmacologic effectiveness of an agent remains consistent in most studies, the placebo effect can vary widely. Dramatic differences have been reported depending on location—e.g., a placebo healing rate for ulcer treatment of 62% in Germany compared to 17% in Denmark and the Netherlands. Moerman (2002) discovered that placebo effectiveness ranged from 10-90%. His findings suggest that effective use of the placebo effect can lead to profound healing.

Believing you are taking care of yourself is part of the cure, so it should not be surprising that compliance itself, and knowing that you are conscientiously following instructions, should make a difference. We naturally expect a drug to be more effective with increased compliance, but studies show that consistent use, even of a placebo, leads to better outcomes. The Coronary Drug Project examined the use of a lipid-lowering drug versus a placebo. The five-year mortality was approximately the same in both groups. What seemed to have the greater effect was compliance rates. Good adherers (taking at least 80% of their meds, whether the actual drug or the placebo) had a lower mortality rate, 15% less—a remarkable demonstration of the power of expectation itself.

The placebo effect is not something to be feared. By denying or ignoring it, we arbitrarily restrict the practice of medicine. I would like to coin a new phrase—Therapeutic Interventional Potential or TIP—to draw attention to the mind's tremendous capacity to heal. Let us harness the powers of the mind-body connection and consider it a vital aspect of our delivery of care.

CHAPTER EIGHT

The Mystery of Death and Beyond

My exploration of the art of medicine must culminate in a discussion of spirit. Spirit is that which is not verifiable using the five senses or scientific analysis. In the broadest sense, one can describe it as the connection of the individual to something greater. The Hebraic biblical term for spirit is *ruach,* referring to breath or wind. It is not tangible, but it is understood. To explore the realm of spirit, we must rely on individual experiences and narratives. In our technological society, things that cannot be measured are diminished in value, but as I have argued from the beginning, this view is too narrow. We must make room for the individual and give value to personal experience.

Most people have had déjà vu experiences, when a situation feels like something they've already encountered. This is a personal phenomenon and cannot be challenged by the outside observer. Different explanations can be offered, but mystery cannot be denied a seat at the table. Perhaps we are accessing information from a source other than our five senses. There are also stories of people knowing when close relatives or friends have died thousands of miles away, when there was no indication of impending doom. Somehow, the limitations of time and space were transcended. Religious rituals intentionally foster such experiences of transcendence. I have felt the presence of spirit during Indigenous ceremonies when smudging—a purifying ritual involving the burning of sacred herbs—was used to create a sacred space. These experiences were profound, and yet I have no words for them.

It is a waste to dismiss alternative belief systems simply because they do not jibe with our own. We should feel compelled to seek what binds us together rather than what differentiates us. Even our body is a community, containing fewer of its own cells relative to microorganisms (the microbiome). The very energy that fuels us is the result of a partnership—mitochondria, the powerhouse of the cell, originated from free-living bacteria that our cells incorporated. We are so used to the idea of the individual as a distinct, autonomous being, it can be hard to acknowledge such partnerships. Focused on lines of demarcation, we cannot see the interdependence, the way people can become blind to the presence of a gorilla when they are told to focus on counting.

The boundaries separating us are not as definitive as we assume, and there is good reason to question the particulate idea of individual life, making room for a greater sense of continuity. The Princeton Engineering Anomalies Research Lab explored nonlocal effects for over thirty years, with much of the research funded by the US Department of Defense (in competition with Russia, who was also actively exploring the field). The studies were sophisticated, including one by the Global Consciousness Project that involved placing random number generating computers around the world and analyzing the randomness of the output over years. Cataclysmic events in the world, such as 9/11, appeared to lead to mathematically analyzable deviations from randomness. These studies can be criticized, but a project that lasts for almost thirty years at a prestigious university merits attention.

The Institute of Noetic Sciences has published a significant number of studies and meta-analyses providing statistical proof of the ability of individuals to receive and obtain information beyond what is available to the five senses. These studies are not always consistent, but this is the case also with RCTs that pass muster. And I do not believe that RCTs are the only justification for belief. In general, this area of spiritual phenomena lies beyond the scope of standard research, and individual stories and experiences may still be our best source of information.

A case that has always fascinated me is that of Claire Sylvia, an adult woman who received a heart-lung transplant using the organs of a teenager who died in a motorcycle accident. Post-surgery, she developed a taste for beer and chicken nuggets, only later discovering that these were foods that the teenager had enjoyed. This is just one of many cases that offer a glimpse into our interconnectedness. No matter how we choose to interpret them, we can remain open to the possibilities. For myself, the idea that I and my patient were part of a broader and, to some extent, unfathomable unity was inspiring. Without a doubt, it improved my care. It fostered feelings of profound humility and compassion, and it transformed my relationship to patients and friends who were dying.

The more I contemplated the mystery of death, the more I saw it as a transition, a window onto a larger sphere of existence. Buddhism, which has been my personal avenue of exploration, describes various liminal states after the consciousness has separated from the physical body. *The Tibetan Book of Living and Dying*, by Sogyal Rinpoche, is a classic text detailing the various bardos, or phases of existence between death and rebirth. I have also learned about *delogs*, individuals usually from the Tibetan culture who have supposedly died and come back to life, days or weeks after death, to relate their experiences. One well-documented story comes from Dawa Drolma, who would go in and out of near-death experiences in a regular, planned manner. She told of being given information during her sojourn in the afterlife, enabling her at one point to locate buried coins known only to someone who was already deceased. The veracity of these accounts is difficult to ascertain, and in a science-based culture, the underlying beliefs can be hard to fathom, but they can serve to broaden the conversation about end of life and what it means. Currently, this conversation is far too limited.

In the West, there are plenty of accounts that can help foster discussion. Dr. Jeffrey Long (2011) details over 3,000 narratives of near-death experiences, codifying them according to recurring themes and presentations that range across cultures, belief systems, and ages. The neurosurgeon Allan Hamilton (2009) presents the case of Pam

Reynolds, who had a brain aneurysm that required surgery with no blood flow—a state of hypothermic cardiac arrest. She was "dead" with no heartbeat or respiration. Medical monitoring confirmed this morbid state. After a successful surgery, she had quite a story to tell. She was aware of hovering over the operating table and then approaching a tunnel of light where she felt the presence of relatives—they were blocking her departure. Reentering her body felt like "plunging into a pool of ice." She recalled hearing one of the surgeons remarking that her arteries were too small for the cardiac bypass tubing, and she could identify the music playing—"Hotel California." All observations were verified by the surgical team. Of course, there are various hypotheses explaining how she knew what was occurring while flatlined. Ultimately, the believers and the skeptics are entitled to their interpretations. But personally, I find in her account and others much food for thought and contemplation. The possibility of a consciousness that is separate from the body will not be easily resolved. My intention is not to revise anyone's personal beliefs. Rather, my aim is to broaden the realm of exploration.

Death is often considered, by doctors and lay people alike, a thing to be feared and fought. The truth is, we know very little about it. What lies beyond is a mystery. If death is no longer something to be avoided at all costs, we can start thinking of it as a transition to navigate. Doctors are often intimately involved with their patients' approach to death, and no matter their specific beliefs, they can play a role whose importance is difficult to overestimate. Entering into a more open-minded relationship with death, we can act with more foresight, reverence, and skill. Elizabeth Kubler Ross' seminal work, *On Death and Dying,* made us all aware of the importance of understanding and appreciating end-of-life issues. Dr. Rachel Naomi Remen has written extensively about the relationships between family and the dying patient. The need for community and support during the final hours of life is of paramount importance to both the dying and living.

It is natural that doctors should focus on prolonging their patients' lives, but approaching death requires a different mentality, and the more mindful doctors are of what is needed, the more sacred the transition can become for everyone involved. I myself have had the great privilege of participating in a number of such transitions, and they have left me feeling full of awe and reverence.

Shakespeare's Hamlet opines, "There are more things in heaven and earth, Horatio, than are dreamt of in your philosophy." If we can open our minds, then death can become so much more than a mere cessation. And if the sanctity and somber awesomeness of death can be recognized unequivocally, then a truly magnificent realm of experience awaits us in the here and now.

> To attain knowledge, add things every day.
> To attain wisdom, remove things every day.
> Lao-Tzu

I'd like now to share with you some of my personal experiences— of people dying with dignity, surrounded by love.

JENNY

A woman in her sixties was diagnosed with a metastatic adrenal tumor. I was consulted because of Cushing's syndrome, uncontrolled cortisol production leading to diabetes, hypertension, and other metabolic abnormalities. She came into the office with her devoted husband to map out a plan for a situation that was difficult to manage. There were treatment protocols, but all had problems and the territory was unclear. None of my efforts was focused on eradication of the tumor; my task was the alleviation of a hormonal imbalance wreaking havoc on the body. The oncologists had little to offer to cure the cancer without making her life even more miserable. We did make headway controlling the hormonal imbalance, but my medications were having less effect as the cancer grew.

I developed a close relationship with her and her husband, and there was great mutual respect. I felt that Jenny was an extraordinary woman who was very clear as to what was happening and, at the same time, trying to lead as normal a life as possible. Her husband gave her unswerving support and wanted to do everything he could to promote her emotional and physical comfort. They had complete confidence in my decisions and eventually decided only to see me. This was a heavy burden for me to handle, and I would spend big chunks of time learning what other options she had and making sure I was doing the best for her. I discussed her case with an oncologist specialist who had a lot of experience with this type of adrenal cancer. It was decided that they should go down to Texas to explore some options there. Upon their return, they let me know that there were no other reasonable scenarios, and they simply wanted to continue having me involved in her total care.

I stayed in touch with the oncologist, but the buck stopped with me regarding any decision. This included any prognosis as to how long she had before expiring. Her potassium became difficult to manage despite maximum treatment, and her blood sugars were requiring increasing amounts of insulin. Jenny asked to be admitted to the hospital for further care. She definitely had enough problems and symptoms to be admitted. Over the next 48 hours, she improved just slightly, and I knew that continued hospitalization would not stem her decline. I talked about stopping treatments and turning to hospice and comfort care. Jenny wanted to stay in the hospital instead of going home because she felt she would be a burden on her family. I knew her husband well and could not believe that to be true. I called her husband, and we had a family conference the next day. Everyone's feelings and desires were expressed, and Jenny realized that love and concern for her well-being dictated that she spend her last waking hours with her family in her home. She expired three days later, surrounded by her family and no longer on any medical regimen. In the end, the bonds of love and interconnection had only grown stronger. It was a beautiful experience of a passage that was meaningful, the patient surrounded by love.

HOWARD

Howard, my father-in-law, lived in North Dakota most of the year and in Arizona during the winter. He was an affable man with the gift of the gab and loved being around people and family. As he entered his mid-eighties, he declined significantly with emphysema caused by smoking as well as failing eyesight and hearing. His days of duck hunting were over, and he was becoming increasingly depressed. Ongoing respiratory complaints led to a chest X-ray, which showed a small spot on the lung. The immediate concern was squamous cell cancer.

I had been involved from afar as a medical advisor for health matters. My suggestion was to wait with surgery, which was very risky, and instead monitor the spot. Other options would be a skinny needle biopsy, but there was a great risk of deflating the lung. The decision was made to go ahead with surgery. His postoperative course was rocky, with a prolonged need for ventilator support. Oddly, the spot on his lung turned out to be a melanoma without any primary source being found elsewhere (there are no melanin-producing cells in the lungs). Surgery is never performed on tumors resulting from metastasis.

I never discussed this with him when I flew to North Dakota to see him in the ICU. I had been told by my wife that he was barely responsive, and a decision had to be made to either stop ventilator support or perform a tracheotomy. I had always had a good relationship with Howard, and we respected each other a lot even though there were major cultural differences. When I entered his room and my wife announced my arrival, he opened his eyes and immediately gave me a thumbs-up. I understood that my presence was like the cavalry coming to rescue him. He became very focused and attentive as I explained that if he didn't start breathing better on his own and put effort into every breath, he would need another surgery, which none of us wanted. He appeared to salute me and immediately went to work on learning to breathe without a machine. By the end of the day, he was off the ventilator.

Unfortunately, the surgery had severely decreased his pulmonary reserves, so he left the hospital after several days in a precarious state. His baseline vision and hearing were also decreased. His quality of life, in short, was horrible. Within a week of discharge, he was back in the hospital with respiratory issues. He refused reintubation and was discharged the next day to go home to die. All of his family, as far away as Costa Rica, were able to be with him as he gradually entered a coma and expired. His family and wife respected his wishes for a cessation of treatment. Howard died with dignity and love, after a life well-lived.

ROBERT

Robert was my best friend from age ten to eighteen. We were more like brothers since he was the only child of parents who weren't around much, and he spent many hours at my house. For several decades during our adult life, we were not in contact, but when we finally did meet again, the closeness that we'd enjoyed in the past reemerged seamlessly. Robert was a successful L.A. lawyer in the entertainment field and surrounded by people who cared a lot about him.

Unfortunately, he developed a very aggressive lymphoma that was not responding to sophisticated treatment management. Even with all the extremely respected specialists taking care of him, Robert turned to me for counsel regarding every medical regimen that was proposed, and as complications piled up and his quality of life dwindled, he wanted me to be the person to tell him enough was enough and that treatments would only perpetuate his pain and suffering. That time arrived, and he was completely peaceful, surrounded by a mélange of human beings who had the utmost love and respect for him.

I flew down from Seattle to be with him for this last time. He was on a hospital bed in his house, basically unclothed, with a sheet wrapped around his loins. His arms were extended in an almost Christ-like pose. Nearly comatose, he nonetheless seemed aware of my presence. After two days, I had to leave to go back to work. Early the next morning, I was meditating as I usually do when I wake up. There was a bright, diffused light present, and the atmosphere was joyful, almost playful. Right after finishing my meditation, there was a message on my cell from Robert's daughter that he had passed.

As I reflected during the course of the day on my experiences with Robert, a particular visit struck me. We had gone to the LA County Museum of Art, where there was an exhibit by James Turrell, a light installation artist. Together, we entered a small enclosure full of bright, white light—it felt like we were entering another dimension. Previously, I had never had a white light visualization during a meditation. Was it a foreshadowing, perhaps a parting goodbye, or was I just taking comfort in happenstance?

In the accounts that follow, I describe my experiences of being present when the person draws their last breath. What transpired (which etymologically means "breathe through") was suffused with an atmosphere of mystery.

JIM

Jim (I've given him a fictitious name to protect his privacy) was a man in his sixties who had been treated for several years in an intermittent fashion for diabetes and its complications, with minimal compliance. He made an appointment with me for discomfort in his right leg. That was an understatement of the problem. I had hardly entered the exam room before I became aware of a putrefying stench. The patient was neither panicked nor overly concerned, even though his right leg showed advanced gangrene. I immediately admitted him to the hospital for an amputation and IV antibiotic treatment. His prognosis was grim with multiple diabetic complications, including renal failure, peripheral vascular disease, and coronary artery disease. It was amazing that he was still alive after surgery. Every day, his condition worsened. He was in the hospital in the early 1980s when hospice was not an option.

It was a lonely time since no family came to visit, but he did not seem to mind. No emotions of anger or sadness were evident. There was just the inexorable course of his deterioration. Eventually, all means of support, including IVs, were stopped, and he slipped into a coma. The nurses became frantic over their inability to get a blood pressure reading or feel a pulse. There were some shallow breaths but no other signs of life. At least, there was no evidence of discomfort or pain. It was difficult for the nurses to accept the lack of vital signs, and they would call me every three or four hours, wanting to know what to do. At the end of the day, while I was examining him and noting still some shallow, regular breaths emanating from his mouth, an unusual thought entered my mind: *Maybe, he doesn't know that he can let go of his life.* He did not appear to have much insight into what was happening to his ravaged body. I decided to take his hand in mine and say softly to him that he could die and stop trying to live any longer. No sooner had I said those words than his breathing stopped, and he developed the pallor of death. I have always wondered if my communication with him made a difference. The patient was definitely comatose according to physical examination. But perhaps he heard me and understood. Not only that, it seemed that he had enough control to end his body's struggle in a hopeless cause. Many might say it was a coincidence, but for me, it was an experience of mystery and awe.

BETTY

My mother-in-law was a quiet, accomplished housewife from North Dakota who took adversity in stride. She had significant health problems, going all the way back to the herniated disc she got during her final pregnancy (the one resulting in the birth of my wife), for which she underwent one of the first discectomies, performed at the Mayo Clinic. She had breast cancer when she was in her early seventies and, after a mastectomy, took tamoxifen, an anti-estrogen, for five years. During this time, she also had a melanoma on her leg excised. She handled these serious medical conditions without any overt anxiety. She was never intrusive or demanding, and she adapted well to life without Howard. Her days were filled with crafts, cooking, and family activities with her children and grandchildren. Winters she spent in Arizona, directing a Sweet Adeline chorus, part of an international organization of women singing four-part acapella with choreographed performances. During one of her sessions with the chorus, she suffered a stroke, with aphasia and paralysis. Her independent lifestyle had come to an end, and my wife brought her to a center with tiered care where she could get rehab and socialize. Melanie, who was also a Sweet Adeline, spent hours encouraging her mother to sing, and it was this gift that helped her to regain her speech. Unfortunately, her right hemiplegia kept her confined to a wheelchair. Then, the breast cancer reappeared, ten years after her initial diagnosis.

I had always been an important resource for her as she navigated her various medical problems, but after I talked to her about her enlarged liver, which was probably a recurrence of her breast cancer, she would see no doctor but me. I tried to talk to her about other options and other specialists, but Betty was not interested, at one time simply turning to my wife to ask if she was going to die.

As Betty's health deteriorated, she continued to emanate a sense of undeterred stateliness. I had discussed with her the fact that she had a liver metastasis that we weren't going to examine or treat further, and this elicited no questions. Her general demeanor was peaceful, and she was unperturbed by her health problems. I gave her medication to decrease the toxins building up due to her failing liver so that she could be alert enough to interact with her daughter. Both of them benefitted from their ongoing communication. Luckily, she did not suffer significant discomfort or pain. As she became increasingly jaundiced, I suggested that we stop the lactulose, which was becoming less effective in keeping her alert. Her son and daughter-in-law flew in from Costa Rica. Unfortunately, I had an important conference to attend and had to leave. I told Betty, who was comfortable but not responsive to conversation, that I was happy she was resting comfortably, surrounded by loving family. I would be gone for three days and return to her bedside as soon as the plane landed. I did not expect her to be alive when I returned.

Betty was still breathing when I returned to Seattle. No one can ever know for certain when a person will expire, but I was surprised that her body was still endowed with life. I walked into her room in the care center where she was surrounded by family and took her hand, saying how glad I was to be back to see her again. I hoped that she was comfortable. Her breathing was slow but regular, and she had a palpable pulse but showed no signs of outer awareness. It was decided that I would go out to get some food with my brother-in-law and his wife while Melanie stayed with her mother. Any changes in Betty's physical status would be immediately conveyed to us by cellphone. About half an hour after we left, Melanie called, and we returned to Betty's bedside. She was having irregular breathing and some death rattles. We held hands together and laid them on Betty. In her passing, she was as sublimely peaceful as she had been in life. I could not get the thought out of my head that Betty did not want to pass until I returned. We did have a good relationship, but did she really need me there before she expired? My gut feeling was that, at some level, she wanted me to be included with the other loving people that were with her. She always tried to make everyone feel welcomed. At her death, there was a sense of spiritual union present that needed no formal religious practice to sanctify it.

HARRY

My dad was, as I mentioned, a general practitioner adored by his patients in the Bronx. He was a mensch who would work up to seven days a week and did house calls. After retiring, he played a daily Scrabble game with his wife, voraciously read books from the library, and worked on a stamp collection. My dad was ninety-three when my mother died from lung cancer, and he sold his condo and moved in with my sister, who absolutely doted on him. He got an iPad and became an online Scrabble addict. Very often, elderly spouses die within a year of each other, but not my dad. He adapted to his new life easily.

Unfortunately, my kind, sweet sister was diagnosed with metastatic ovarian cancer that limited her ability to take care of our dad. Luckily, she had an initial, almost miraculous response to surgery and chemotherapy, resulting in no evidence of cancer on scans. Ultimately, she had a recurrence and was back on chemotherapy. Meanwhile, my dad developed an upper respiratory infection. Because of the immuno-compromised state of my sister under treatment, it was decided that my dad would be admitted to the hospital. He was ninety-six with a sharp mind but an increasingly frail body, compromised by both aortic stenosis and controlled Crohn's disease. His body started to unravel in the hospital with complications from antibiotic use as well as generalized weakness, leading to difficulty swallowing and refusal to eat. He was getting IV fluids for basic fluid replacement and subsistence nutritional support. I made the trip to New Jersey from Seattle to be with him and to determine the best course of action, heeding the input and advice of his doctors.

I encouraged him to eat the soft diet provided but did not have much success. NG tube feedings were initiated to bolster his nutritional status, but this is an approach that can only be continued for so long. My inclination was not to pursue aggressive treatment since he was looking very frail, and with my sister getting chemotherapy, there was no chance of him returning to her house if he recovered. He would end up in a nursing facility that could not provide him the loving care to which he was accustomed. I was interested in my dad dying with dignity and in peace, and I talked to him about stopping nutritional support and going on hospice.

My dad wavered in his decision and finally chose to have a gastrostomy tube inserted directly into his stomach for long-term nutritional support. He had a postoperative bleed and continued to go downhill. Despite his dire condition, he always found some energy to spend time playing Scrabble online.

The day before his death, my dad had his final Scrabble victory against my wife, Melanie. His final day started in the usual manner. I entered his hospital room and parted the curtain surrounding his bed. The two nursing aides were giving him a hand bath. He looked at me and put his hand out, beckoning me to take hold of it. I did, and that was his last breath. No pain, no struggle.

Months later, I was reflecting on that last moment of us holding hands and realized that a photo had immortalized that gesture two years earlier. Melanie had just finished a Shutterfly album commemorating our lives as fathers, with photos of myself with my sons, and of my father with me. The next to last photo was taken from behind, as my dad and I were walking through the atrium of the Chihuly museum in Seattle. The space, with its glass dome, was airy and filled with light, and we were walking through the light together, holding hands. Melanie had even included a cropped insert of just our hands.

MELANIE

I wonder if this part is being written more for my own needs than for a reader's benefit. Perhaps, by recounting the most intense part of my life, I will convey something of meaning or significance.

My wife had a possible premonition of her cancer when, during a glass bowl sound vibration session, she felt weighted down. The intent of the session was to promote calmness with healing energies. In retrospect, it might have been a diagnostic test, hinting at ominous changes. It was about two months later that her illness was diagnosed. Melanie was very active in the Sweet Adeline organization as a performer, choreographer, and national/international judge. In the year 2014, her travel schedule was heavy; she'd come home for a week, only to leave the week after. The regimen was tiring but satisfying, so no big complaints. But she developed a cough, which was worse each time she returned. I decided to suspend my role as husband and step into that of physician. I examined her throat, palpated her neck, and took out a stethoscope to listen to her lungs. No breath sounds on the right side of her chest and dullness to percussion— very concerning. She needed a chest X-ray right away.

A privilege of being a physician is being able to bypass the usual channels to get medical help. The next morning, Melanie had an X-ray, which showed a whiteout of the right lung field. I immediately took her to my pulmonologist colleague, who agreed that a CAT scan was needed with drainage of pleural fluid. As yet, I had no desire to wring my hands with worry and anxiety. I just needed information. The radiologists removed over 1.5 liters of fluid, and the CAT scan showed a mass with lymph node enlargement. Melanie and I were facing a diagnosis of metastatic lung cancer. I was blessed with knowing how the medical system works and was able to accelerate the process of diagnosis, which even then was not easy or straight-forward. Imaging is one part, but tissue is the ultimate piece in the puzzle. Different cancers of the lung require different treatments. Very quickly, we had a slew of specialists involved in determining the next step of this journey. The pulmonologist referred us to a thoracic surgeon to consider doing a pleural biopsy to get a diagnosis, as well as a pleurodesis, a procedure that adheres the lung to the chest wall so that fluid cannot accumulate in that now obliterated space. At the same time, we made an appointment to see an oncologist, Dr. Henry Kaplan, a physician respected by my peers. The thoracic surgeon wanted to set up surgery immediately while the oncologist did not want an invasive action to be done so soon. His idea was to do a biopsy via bronchoscopy and monitor how fast fluid was reaccumulat-ing before performing an invasive procedure that causes pain, carries the risk of complications, and, moreover, may not even be successful if no pleural mass is found to biopsy. Most lay people would have chosen the more invasive route. We opted for the slower and more deliberate approach.

In my discussion of the placebo effect, I noted that patients often feel better with a more invasive approach. It is human nature. I thought that I was taking the more rational approach, and my deci-sion was reinforced by the very experienced and esteemed oncologist. In retrospect, the surgical direction might well have been better for Melanie, with less discomfort and complications. The bronchoscopy biopsy was performed, with the malignant effusion reaccumulating quickly, requiring an outpatient drainage of the fluid. In three days, another drainage was needed and a pleurX tube was inserted into the pleural space so that I could do further drainages at home. If we had done the pleurodesis, the need for ongoing drainage might have been avoided. To make matters worse, the pleurX site developed a bacterial staphylococcus infection. Another reason for doing the bronchoscopy was that there would be no need to wait for the surgery site to heal before chemotherapy. It turns out that we did not save any time by not doing surgery since results took ten days to come back anyway.

Finally, we got the results of the biopsy with the diagnosis of adeno-carcinoma of the lung, for which chemotherapy has a poor record.

The good news, relatively speaking, was that the tumor had a marker that allowed Melanie to be a candidate for a biologic, which targeted her tumor directly and had shown some promising results. The drug was Tarceva, a pill taken once a day. One avoids the significant side effects of chemotherapy, but there are still potential negative reactions, among them ageusia, the loss of the sense of taste, which sounded unpleasant but not horrendous. It turned out to be hell. For the rest of her life, Melanie was unable to taste food, with the progressive problem of eating less and less. What was worse, the drug did not stop the progression of the cancer. It did not work. Why not, when Melanie fitted the criteria to a tee? Probably because cancer is a dynamic process that can morph into other forms via mutation, outwitting science. The time had arrived for a prescribed regimen of chemotherapy.

Cancer care can be a roller coaster of highs and lows. It is important to strap yourself in and look for moments of solace, distraction, and connection to others. I was Melanie's main support and was able to devote all my time to her. I had just retired from my practice, and my research center was going well, requiring minimal involvement. We had been married for thirty years and were used to discussing issues in an open and intimate fashion. Now, we would be proceeding down a path of even deeper meaning and closeness. It was a privilege for me to be able to take care of her, even though the circumstances were dismal.

Melanie had always been a very independent woman whose modus operandi was taking care of others. To my sons' friends, even when they were adults, she was Mama Melanie and an important resource. She played various roles in the Sweet Adelines and affected the lives of thousands of women. Now, she would have to let me be her caretaker, and her role would be to receive love and care from others.

As soon as she was given the diagnosis, Melanie cancelled her extensive responsibilities with the Sweet Adelines and devoted herself to cancer management. Life did not stop, of course, and we had close friends with whom we maintained contact. One couple were doctors and contributed to medical care and decision-making. Another couple would arrange small social gatherings with a coterie of friends for a meal that included whatever Melanie cared to eat. Those affairs would soon come to an end since Melanie became averse to eating. With other friends, we had bridge nights. As I mentioned earlier, social contact is a vital part of healthcare regimens. Eventually, however, even those activities ceased.

Surprisingly, she tolerated chemo well. The ever-present loss of taste remained a big problem. We never discussed prognosis, as I wanted to keep a positive attitude regarding the treatment regimen. Only later did I learn that Melanie was planning for her demise, before chemo even began, by recording her thoughts, feelings, and hopes for our sons and myself, to be read after she passed. She gave no hint of knowing that all the efforts to prolong her life would be unsuccessful.

Melanie underwent the chemo and the debilitating course of her cancer because we had learned that our older son and his wife were expecting a child, and she wanted to be present for the birth and look presentable. As soon as she knew she was starting chemo, she went to a wig maker to have a wig made from her own hair. (Ironically, Melanie never lost her stubble of hair during chemo.) When the wig was done, we had to go immediately to her hair stylist to shape the hair to her specifications. Ultimately, Melanie would only wear this wig a single time when we went to a wedding. She did not want to garner any attention and distract from the bride. Otherwise, her head gear consisted of a variety of colorful scarves.

Her treatment regimen revolved around chemo, which had a mildly positive effect, and various alternative treatments to help symptoms and improve her general well-being. Melanie was not a big believer in alternative therapies, but with my prodding, she consented to give them a try. Acupuncture did not help at all, but energy work and healing at a distance had some beneficial effects on her general outlook. CBD was tried to stimulate her appetite but had no effect. Eventually, she developed severe back pain and needed conventional pain medication, but she often got more relief from Arnica, an herbal preparation. The skillful use of small needles in her back (dry needling) also helped. These alternative pain-relieving therapies were always appreciated since Melanie did not tolerate conventional opioids well.

The last couple of months leading to hospice were a time of poignancy and simplicity. The deep connection between us was palpable, without the need for words to affirm it. I would be scurrying around the place, making her a shake, cleaning the house, making sure she was comfortable. Melanie would look up at me, patting the couch next to her, and say, "Just be my friend and be with me." The TV would be on a lot to distract her. She loved to watch the Mariners play baseball. In the past, she'd had a mild interest in baseball; now she became a fanatic. Together, we watched the complete DVD series of *Little House on the Prairie*, a favorite of hers as she grew up in North Dakota. Throughout her illness, there were the electronic communications that took hours of her day. Facebook became an important part of her support system. Melanie had always been gregarious and had an extensive group of Facebook friends, the greatest number being Sweet Adelines. Her followers were over a thousand, and if they did not get frequent posts from her, they'd get in touch with me to find out what was happening. Her contacts were global—in Sweden, England, New Zealand, and Australia—as well as scattered across the United States. Occasionally, a well-meaning woman would post a response to which Melanie reacted negatively, prompting an immediate unfriending. Another woman wrote from Down Under that people were thinking of Melanie 24 hours a day because somewhere in the world, there was always someone who was up. Melanie knew how to maintain a support system that felt right, separating the seed from the chaff. Technology has its benefits, connecting people in meaningful ways.

During the last month of her life, she commented that she was looking like a cancer patient, gaunt with only a stubble of hair. The back pain got worse, and imaging showed a metastasis. To me, the game was over, and all I wanted for her was comfort care. However, Melanie opted for radiation treatment to shrink the tumor in the spine. It became increasingly difficult to get her to her oncologist and the radiation center, and yet she persevered. Why did she tolerate this agony? She wanted to see the birth of her granddaughter.

Her weakness increased, and she was unable to eat. A precipitous drop in her sodium level, a recurrent problem, sent her to the hospital. I had been talking to Melanie in earnest about comfort care. It was hard to see her suffer as her body spiraled into an uncontrollable mess. Metabolically, Melanie was stabilized with IV treatment, but to maintain any semblance of life, she would need TPN through the port that was being used for her chemo. Initially, she was adamant about getting complete nutritional support. I spoke with the oncologist about my concerns around prolonging her downhill course for minimum gain. We decided to provide her with our best estimation of what her time course would be, with and without TPN, so she could make an informed decision. As soon as she heard that TPN might give her only an extra two weeks of life and there was no chance of her surviving an extra three months to see the birth of her granddaughter, Melanie looked at me and said, "Let's go home." So, we did. I set up hospice support and let our two sons and her brother and sister know.

Melanie was fine with being on hospice but did not realize that she was going to die at home. When we talked about getting a hospital bed in the house, she was astonished. "I will not die at home!" Why? She did not want the pall of death to permeate our home, creating negative associations for me and our sons. We had a meeting, and the whole family pleaded with her, explaining that we wanted to be with her every moment we could and that our home would be a sanctuary for us and hopefully for her as well. Melanie realized the full extent of our love and understood that being separated while she took the final steps of her journey was not an option.

Hospice is about intimate, intense relationships with a vulnerable population. Unfortunately, the industrial complex has a different emphasis. I was not quite prepared for the slew of paperwork and at times overwhelming, bureaucratic procedures. There was an intake person, then a logistics person, and finally the hospice nurse. When Melanie's back pain grew worse, I requested a patient-controlled analgesia. It should have been simple and quick, but first Melanie had to be evaluated, then the medicine had to be delivered, then the nurse had to return to set it up. I won't go on, except to say that the delays were absurd and extremely frustrating. This does not take away from my esteem for the care rendered by hospice workers or my respect for hospice itself, an invaluable institution.

Regardless, the final scene of the last act was unfolding. All the aspirations and trials and tribulations were now part of the past. My only intentions were for a smooth transition to finality. While Melanie was still conscious and alert, the family assembled. Melanie's brother Steve and his wife Teresita flew in from Costa Rica and her sister Jan arrived from Minnesota. My sons were already holding vigil.

Melanie was weak and had told me several months earlier that I should check in with her when company was present in case she needed rest and the guests should be asked to leave. Her final conscious gathering of her family was a tour de force, a party atmosphere peeking out from the solemnity of the occasion. Steve, her older brother by seven years, broke the ice by sharing letters that he had saved from Melanie when he first moved to Costa Rica, over forty years before. The younger sister was reading him the riot act on who he should be and what he should do—true impertinence. Everyone was entertained, hearing the words that Melanie had written so long ago, but which defined so well the way she had led her life—direct, forthright, caring. Melanie was smiling but could not say much because of weakness. I whispered in her ear whether I should ask everyone to leave so she could rest. Melanie summoned up some hidden strength and, looking into my eyes, said, "This is my party and I love it."

The next morning, she was semi-comatose and no longer interacting. Her patient-controlled analgesia was working fine, and she appeared comfortable. A windstorm was whipping through the trees, and then the lights went out. It was dusk, and we set up candles around her bed. Melanie loved candles and would often bring them on our trips. It was a fitting touch to have her flooded with candlelight. I felt that she was putting together her last piece of choreography, and the solemnity of the moment flickered with mystery and awe. Then the electricity came back on, and all that was left was for her to pass on. In the early morning hours, she expired, surrounded by her two grown boys and me. Tears of loss and grief were shed, but the end had transpired with dignity and nobility, pervaded by love.

CLOSING THOUGHTS

"I am not just a statistic" is the cry of those who feel that the delivery of high-quality care has become sterile and clinical. My most fervent hope is for the integration of modern, evidence-based medicine with a more holistic approach, a melding of the rock-solid superstructure of a technological age with the ethereal qualities of awe and the mystery of life. Life perceived as a whole, an entity that cannot be divided into its parts, is sacrosanct. If our goal is to alleviate suffering and pain, other belief systems and therapeutic methods must be considered. Pharmaceuticals have been a boon, as have life-saving advances in healthcare technology. Supported by clinical trials, they are a significant piece of the picture, but how big a piece? That is the crucial question. To focus on this one realm as if it represented the whole, choosing to ignore variables that are often of greater significance, is to steer an arbitrary course and cut ourselves off from some of the most powerful wellsprings of good health.

Above all, let us recognize what lies at the heart of healthcare: the patient-doctor relationship. Words matter as well as body language and a presence that is pervasive, radiating concern, compassion, and yes, even love for the individual. The goal is to be authentic and in touch with our emotional side as well as our intellect. When a patient goes to Lourdes, perhaps it is the force of compassion and love that heals more than the waters. And in the case of faith healing, perhaps it is the intentions and attentions of the healer and broader community that are the wellspring. To fulfill our potential, we must cultivate not just the science of medicine but the art.

A kaleidoscope of facts and figures whirls in the physician's brain, but they are surrounded by ambiguity and uncertainty in a universe whose complex interconnectivity surpasses description. The practice of medicine requires humility and collaboration, listening with heart and heeding inner wisdom. The focus is not the drug. Nor is it simply curing the patient. It is being with the patient, in the profoundest way, no matter the situation or ultimate outcome.

In the words of T.S. Eliot,

> We shall not cease from exploration,
> And the end of all our exploring,
> Will be to arrive where we started
> And know the place for the first time.

In the end, love and connection are all that count. May this book be like a sand mandala, created with meticulous care and then dissolving, leaving only an imprint on the mind and some suggestion, slight though it may be, of our universal destination.

HOMAGE

The original impetus to write this book came from my desire to thank my patients for being a part of my life and sharing with me the rich diversity of their human experience—from deep grief to lighthearted silliness. I have kept the one hundred or so cards and letters of appreciation that they wrote for my retirement. Their reflections run the gamut from simple appreciation to expressions of intimate connection. They offer a fair portrayal of what I wanted to accomplish in my medical career. Reading these words, I can visualize the various patients who wrote them. It brings me to tears to appreciate the effect I had on their lives. I want to let them know how profoundly they helped me to become a better clinician and person.

Regarding the book itself, I would like to acknowledge Karin de Weille, a writing consultant and editor who was intimately involved in its development and fulfillment. Not only did she give good technical advice, she was a muse helping to bring my message to fruition.

GLOSSARY OF TERMS
AND ABBREVIATIONS

AA – Alcoholics Anonymous

AAFP – American Academy of Family Physicians

ACC/AHA – American College of Cardiology/
American Heart Association

ACCORD – Action and Control of Cardiovascular Risk in Diabetes

AI – Artificial Intelligence

AL-ANON – Alcoholics Anonymous

ALLHAT – Antihypertensive and Lipid Lowering to Prevent Heart
Attack Trial

AMPM/USDA – Automated Multiple Pass Method
(collection dietary recall)

ASCVD – Arteriosclerotic Cardiovascular Disease

BMD – Bone Mineral Density

BP – Blood Pressure

CAD – Coronary Artery Disease

CAT scan or CT – Computed Axial Tomography

CBD – Cannabidiol (cannabis extract)

COVID – Coronavirus Disease

DBP – Diastolic Blood Pressure (the second number)

DCCT – Diabetes Complication and Control Trial

DKA – Diabetic Ketoacidosis
(insulin deficient state, fatal if untreated)

DNR – Do Not Resuscitate orders

ECMO – Extracorporeal Membrane Oxygenation

EMR – Electronic Medical Record

ER – Emergency Room

FDA – Food and Drug Administration

FRAX – Fracture Risk Assessment Tool

GMO – Genetically Modified Organism

GRADE – Grade of Recommendation, Assessment,
Development, Evaluation

GSK – GlaxoSmithKline, pharmaceutical company

HDL – High Density Lipoprotein (the good cholesterol)

HMR – Health Management Resources
(very low-calorie liquid diet program)

ICU – Intensive Care Unit

IV – Intravenous (tube into a vein to give fluids or medication)

JNC – Joint National Committee
(numerous hypertension guidelines)

LDL – Low Density Lipoprotein (the bad cholesterol)

MRI – Magnetic Resonance Imaging

NHLB – National Heart, Lung, and Blood Institute

NHS – Nurses' Health Study

NIH – National Institute of Health

OBGYN – Obstetrics/Gynecology

PREDIMED – Prevention with Mediterranean Diet
(a Spanish study)

PSA – Prostatic Specific Antigen

R&D – Research and Development
(of medications/pharmaceuticals)

RCT – Randomized Controlled Trial

RECORD – Rosiglitazone Evaluated for Cardiac Outcomes and
Regulation of Glycemia in Diabetes

SBP – Systolic Blood Pressure (the first number)

SOTI – Spinal Osteoporosis Therapeutic Intervention trial

SPRINT – Systolic Blood Pressure Intervention Trial

TPN – Total Parental Nutrition (via IV central line)

TROPOS – Treatment of Peripheral Osteoporosis Study

UGDP – the University Group Diabetes Program

USPS Task Force – United States Protective Services Task Force

USSR – Union of Soviet Socialist Republics

UTI – Urinary Tract Infection

WEIRD – Western, Educated, Industrialized, Rich, and Democratic

WHI – Women's Health Initiative

WORKS CITED

ACCORD Study Group. (2010). Effects of intensive blood-pressure control in type 2 diabetes mellitus. *New England Journal of Medicine, 362*(17), 1575–85.

Achterberg, J. (1985). Imagery in Healing: Shamanism and Modern Medicine. Shambala.

Achterberg, J., Kenner, C., & Lawlis, G. F. (1988). Severe Burn Injury: A Comparison of Relaxation, Imagery, and Biofeedback for Pain Management. *Journal of Mental Imagery, 12*, 71–87.

Ader, R. & Cohen, N. (1975). Behaviorally Conditioned Immunosuppression. *Psychosomatic Medicine, 37*(4), 333–340.

Agarwal, A. & Ioannidis, J. (2019). PREDIMED trial of Mediterranean diet: retracted, republished, still trusted? *British Medical Journal, 364*, 1341. https://doi.org/10.1136/bmj.l341.

ALLHAT Officers and Coordinators for the ALLHAT Collaborative Research Group. (2002, December 18). Major Outcomes in High-risk Hypertensive Patients Randomized to Angiotensin-converting Enzyme Inhibitor or Calcium Channel Blocker vs Diuretic: The Antihypertensive and Lipid-Lowering Treatment to Prevent Heart Attack Trial (ALLHAT). JAMA, *288*(23), 2981–97. https://doi.org/10.1001/jama.288.23.2981.

Anderson, J. & Muhlestein, J. (2004). Antibiotic Trials for Coronary Heart Disease. *Texas Heart Institute Journal, 31*(1), 33–38.

Andrew, R. & Izzo, A. (2017, June). Principles of Pharmacological Research of Nutraceuticals. *British Journal of Pharmacology, 174*(11),1177–1194.

Angell, N. F. (2004). Controversy Concerning the Women's Health Initiative Trial. *Middle East Fertility Society Journal, 9*(1), 84–86.

Anheyer, D., Frawley, J., Koch, A. K., Langhorst, J., Lauche, R., Dobos, G., & Cramer, H. (2017). Herbal Medicines for Gastrointestinal Disorders in Children and Adolescents: A Systematic Review, *Pediatrics, 139*(6), 1–11.

Aubrey, A. (2019, September 30). No Need To Cut Back On Red Meat? Controversial New "Guidelines" Lead To Outrage. www.wgbh.org/news/science-and-technology/2019/09/30/no-need-to-cut-back-on-red-meat-controversial-new-guidelines-lead-to-outrage

Bahl, M., Barzilay, R., Yedida, A., Locascio, N., Yu, L., & Lehman, C. (2017). High-Risk Breast Lesions: A Machine Learning Model to Predict Pathologic Upgrade and Reduce Unnecessary Surgical Excision. *Radiology, 286*(3), 810–818. https://doi.org/10.1148/radiol.2017170549

Bailey, L.W. (2001). A "Little Death": The Near-Death Experience and Tibetan Delogs. *Journal of Near-Death Studies, 19*(3),139–159.

Bailey, R. (2012, January). Who's More Anti-science: Republicans or Democrats? *Reason.* https://reason.com/2011/12/27/whos-more-anti-science-republicans-or-de/

Bartlett, R. H., Andrews, A. F., Toomasian, J. M., Haiduc, N. J., & Gazzaniga, A. B. (1982). Extracorporeal Membrane Oxygenation for Newborn Respiratory Failure: Forty-Five Cases. *Surgery, 92*(2), 425–433.

Bautista, M. C. & Engler, M. M. (2005). The Mediterranean Diet: Is It Cardioprotective? *Progress in Cardiovascular Nursing, 20*(2), 70–76.

Beecher, H. K. (1955). The Powerful Placebo. *JAMA, 159*(17),1602–1606.

Belluz, J. (2019, February 13). This Mediterranean diet study was hugely impactful. The science has fallen apart. https://www.vox.com/science-and-health/2018/6/20/17464906/mediterranean-diet-science-health-predimed

Benedetti, F. (2012). *The Patient's Brain: The Neuroscience behind the Doctor-Patient Relationship.* Oxford University Press.

Benson, H. (1979). *The Mind/Body Effect.* Simon and Schuster.

Bernhard, T. (2010). *How To Be Sick.* Wisdom Publications.

Black, S., Humphrey, J. H., & Niven, J. S. F. (1963). Inhibition of Mantoux Reaction by Direct Suggestion under Hypnosis. *British Medical Journal, 1*(5346), 1649–1652.

Blackburn, H. & Jacob Jr., D. R. (2017). A Study of the Effects of Hypoglycemic Agents on Vascular Complications in Patients with Adult-Onset Diabetes: II. Mortality Results. *International Journal of Epidemiology, 46*(5), 1354–1364. https://doi.org/10.1093/ije/dyw168

Blakeslee, S. (October 13, 1998). Placebos Prove So Powerful Even Experts Are Surprised; New Studies Explore the Brain's Triumph Over Reality. *New York Times*, Section F, page 1.

Blunt, C. J. (2018, July 26). The Parachute Problem: Extracorporeal Life Support and the Demand for Trials. http://cjblunt.com/

Bohm, D. & Peat, F. D. (1987). *Science, Order, and Creativity*. Bantam Books.

Bolland, M. & Grey, A. (2014). A Comparison of Adverse Event and Fracture Efficacy Data for Strontium Ranelate in Regulatory Documents and the Publication Record. *BMJ Open, 4*(10),1–8. https://doi.org/10.1136/bmjopen-2014-005787

Boyko, E. J. (2013). Observational Research—Opportunity and Limitations. *Journal of Diabetes and Its Complications, 27*(6),642–648.

Bruhn, J. G. (1965). An Epidemiological Study of Myocardial Infarctions in an Italian-American Community, *Journal of Chronic Disease,18*, 353–365.

Brush Jr., J. E. (2015). *The Science of the Art of Medicine: A Guide to Medical Reasoning*. Dementi Milestone Publishing.

Buettner, D. (2016). Blue Zones: Lessons from the World's Longest Lived. *American Journal of Lifestyle Medicine, 10*(5), 318–321. https://doi.org/10.1177/1559827616637066

Burton Goldberg Group, compiler. (1994). *Alternative Medicine: The Definitive Guide*. Future Medicine Publishing.

Carlyle, T. (2001). *A Carlyle Reader: Selections from the Writings of Thomas Carlyle*. Cambridge University Press.

Carroll, S. (2017). *The Big Picture*. Dutton.

Catalona, W. J. (1998). Use of the Percentage of Free Prostate-Specific Antigen to Enhance Differentiation of Prostate Cancer from Benign Prostatic Disease: A Prospective Multicenter Clinical Trial. *JAMA, 279*(19), 1542–1547. https://doi.org/ 10.1001/jama.279.19.1542

Chablis, C. & Daniel Simons. (1999). The Invisible Gorilla. http://theinvisiblegorilla.com/gorilla_experiment.html

Chan, K., Qin, L., Lau, M., Woo, J., Au, S., Choy, W., Lee, K., & Lee, S. (2004). A Randomized, Prospective Study of the Effects of Tai Chi Chun Exercise on Bone Mineral Density in Postmenopausal Women. *Archives of Physical Medicine and Rehabilitation, 85*(5), 717–22. https://doi.org/10.1016/j.apmr.2003.08.091.n

Chou, R., Dana, T., Blazina, I., Daeges, M., & Jeanne, T. (2016). Statins for Prevention of Cardiovascular Disease in Adults: Evidence Report and Systematic Review for the U.S. Preventive Services Task Force. *JAMA, 316*(19), 2008–2024. https://doi.org/10.1001/jama.2015.15629

Christian, B. & Griffiths, T. (2016). *Algorithms to Live By: The Computer Science of Human Decisions*. Henry Holt and Co.

Church, D. (2018). *Mind to Matter: The Astonishing Science of How Your Brain Creates Material Reality.* Hay House.

Cianferotti, L., D'Asta, F., & Brandi, M. L. (2013). A Review on Strontium Ranelate Long-term Antifracture Efficacy in the Treatment of Postmenopausal Osteoporosis. *Therapeutic Advances in Musculoskeletal Disease, 5*(3), 127–139. https://doi.org/ 10.1177/1759720X13483187

Clinician Workgroup on the Integration of Complementary and Alternative Medicine. (2000, January). Issues in Coverage for Complementary and Alternative Medicine Services. Washington State Office of the Insurance Commissioner.

Cobb, L. A., Thomas, G. I., Dillard, D. H., Merendino, K. A., & Bruce, R. A. (1959). An Evaluation of Internal-Mammary-Artery Ligation by a Double-Blind Technic. *New England Journal of Medicine, 260,* 1115–1118. https://doi.org/10.1056/NEJM195905282602204

Cobleigh, M. A., Berris, R. F., Bush, T., Davidson, N. E., Robert, N. J., Sparano, Tormey, D., J. A., & Wood, W. C. (1994). Estrogen Replacement Therapy in Breast Cancer Survivors A Time for Change. *JAMA, 272*(7), 540–545. https://doi.org/10.1001/jama.1994.03520070060039

Colditz, G. A., Stampfer, M. J., Willett, W. C., Hennekens, C. H., Rosner, B., & Speizer, F. E. (1990). Prospective Study of Estrogen Replacement Therapy and Risk of Breast Cancer in Postmenopausal Women. *JAMA, 264*(20), 2648–2653.

Colditz, G. A., Philpott, S. E., & Hankinson, S. E. (2000). The Impact of the Nurses' Health Study on Population Health: Prevention, Translation, and Control. *American Journal of Public Health, 106*(9), 1540–1545. https://doi.org/10.2105/AJPH.2016.303343

Cooper, C., Fox, K., & Borer, J. (2014). Ischemic Events and Use of Strontium Ranelate in Postmenopausal Osteoporosis: A Nested Case-control Study in the CPRD. *Osteoporosis International, 25*(2), 737–745.

Coronary Drug Project Research Group. (1980). Influence of Adherence to Treatment and Response of Cholesterol on Mortality in the Coronary Drug Project. *New England Journal of Medicine, 303*(18), 1038–1041. https://doi.org/10.1056/NEJM198010303031804

Cousins, N. (1979). *Anatomy of an Illness: as Perceived by the Patient.* W.W. Norton& Company.

DeGowin, E. & DeGowin, R. (1976). *Bedside Diagnostic Examination.* Macmillan Publishing Co.

Dhont, M. (2010). History of Oral Contraception. *The European Journal of Contraception and Reproductive Health Care, 15*(2), s12–18. https://doi.org/1 0.3109/13625187.2010.513071

Diabetes Control and Complications Trial Research Group. (1993). The Effect of Intensive Treatment of Diabetes on the Development and Progression of Long-Term Complications in Insulin-Dependent Diabetes Mellitus. *New England Journal of Medicine, 329*, 977–986. https://doi.org/10.1056/ NELM199309303291401

DiMatteo, M. R., Sherbourne, C. D., Hays, D. D., Ordway, L., Kravitz, R. L., McGlynn, E.A., Kaplan, S., & Rogers, W.H. (1993). Physicians' Characteristics Influence Patients' Adherence to Medical Treatment: Results from the Medical Outcome Study. *Health Psychology, 12*(2), 93–102.

Dossey, L. (1999). *Reinventing Medicine: Beyond Mind-Body to a New Era of Healing*. Harper Collins.

Drolma,D. (1995). *Delog Journey to Realms Beyond Death*. (Richard Barron translator). Padma Publishing.

Dubroff, R. (2017). Cholesterol Paradox: A Correlate does not a Surrogate Make. *Evidence-Based Medicine, 22*(1), 15–19. https://doi.org/10.1136/ ebmed-2016-110602

Duffy M.D., T. P. (2011). The Flexner Report—100 Years Later. *Yale Journal of Biology and Medicine, 84*(3): 269–276.

Egbert, L. D., Battit, E., Welch, C. E., & Bartlett, M. K. (1964). Reduction of Postoperative Pain by Encouragement and Instruction of Patients. *New England Journal of Medicine, 270* (16), 1089–1092.

Egnew, T. E. (2014). The Art of Medicine: Seven Skills that Promote Mastery. *Family Practice Management, 21*(4), 25–30.

Egolf, B., Lasker, J., Wolf, S., & Potvin, L. (1992). The Roseto Effect: A 50-Year Comparison of Mortality Rates. *American Journal of Public Health, 82*(8), 1089–1092.

Einstein, A. (2010). *The Ultimate Quotable Einstein* (Alice Calaprice, Ed.). Princeton University Press

Eisenberg, D. (1995). *Encounters with Qi: Exploring Chinese Medicine*. W.W. Norton & Company.

Epstein, R. (2017). *Attending: Medicine, Mindfulness, and Humanity*. Scribner.

Estruch, R., Ros, E., Salas-Salvadó, J., Covas, M., Corella, D., Arós F., Gómez-Gracia, E., Ruiz-Gutiérrez, V., Fiol M., Lapetra, J., Lamuela-Raventos, R.M., & Serra-Majem, L. (2013). Primary Prevention of Cardiovascular Disease with a Mediterranean Diet. *New England Journal of Medicine, 368*:1279–1290.

Fawzy, I., Fawzy, N.W., Hyun, C.S, Elashoff, R., Guthrie D., Fahey, H. Malignant melanoma. Effects of an early structured psychiatric intervention, coping, and affective state on recurrence and survival 6 years later. (1993). *Archives of General Psychiatry, 50* (9), 681–689.

Feinstein, A. R. (1995). Meta-Analysis: Statistical Alchemy for the 21st Century. *Journal of Clinical Epidemiology, 48*(1), 71–79.

Feynman, R. (2010, March 14). To Live with Doubt and Uncertainty. Deeshaa. https://deeshaa.org/2010/03/14/richard-feynman-to-live-with-doubt-and-uncertainty/

Forbes, D. (2013). Blinding: An Essential Component in Decreasing Risk of Bias in Experimental Designs. *Evidence Based Nursing, 16*(3), 70–71.

Foucault, M. (1994). *The Birth of the Clinic: An Archaeology of Medical Perception.* Vintage Books. (Original work published February 11, 1973)

Frawley, D. (1992). *Ayurvedic Healing: A Comprehensive Guide.* Passage Press. (Original work published February 11, 1989)

Frieden, T. R. (2017). Evidence for Health Decision Making- Beyond Randomized, Controlled Trials. *New England Journal of Medicine, 377*, 465–475.

Frost, R. (2015). *The Road Not Taken and Other Poems.* Penguin Books.

Gabriel, S. E., & Normand, S.L.T. (2012). Getting the Methods Right—The Foundation of Patient-Centered Outcomes Research. *New England Journal of Medicine, 367*(9), 787–790.

Gagnier, J.J., Boon, H., Rochon, P., Moher, D., Barnes, J., Bombardier, C., for the CONSORT Group. (2006). Recommendations for Reporting Randomized Controlled Trials of Herbal Interventions: Explanation and Elaboration. *Journal of Clinical Epidemiology, 59*, 1134–1149.

Gawande, A. (2014). *Being Mortal.* Metropolitan Books.

Gawande, A. (2010). *The Checklist Manifesto: How to Get Things Right.* Picador.

Geusens, P., Autier, P., Bonnen, S., Vanhoof, J., Declerk, K., & Raus, J. (2002). The Relationship among History of Falls, Osteoporosis, and Fractures in Post-Menopausal Women. *Archives of Physical Medicine and Rehabilitation, 83*(7), 903–906. https://doi.org/10.1053/apmr.2002.33111.

Golden, H., Bass, E. (2013). Validity of Meta-Analysis in Diabetes: Meta-analysis is an Indispensable Tool in Evidence Synthesis. *Diabetes Care, 36* (10), 3368–3374.

Groopman., J. (2008). *How Doctors Think.* Houghton Mifflin Company.

Groopman, J. (2017, April 3). Is Fat Killing You, or Is Sugar? *The New Yorker.* https://www.newyorker.com/magazine/2017/04/03

Groopman J. & Hartzband., P. (2011). *Your Medical Mind: How to Decide What Is Right for You.* The Penguin Press.

Grundy, S. M. & Stone, N. J. (2019). 2018 Cholesterol Clinical Practice Guidelines: Synopsis of the 2018 American Heart Association/American College of Cardiology/Multisociety Cholesterol Guideline. *Annals of Internal Medicine, 11*(170), 779–783. https://doi.org/10.7326/M19-0365.

Ferré, M., Salas-Salvadó, J., Ros, E., Estruch, R., Corella, D., Fitó, M., Martínez-González, M.A. (2017) The PREDIMED Trial, Mediterranean Diet and Health Outcomes: How Strong is the Evidence. *Nutrition, Metabolism, and Cardiovascular Diseases, 27*(7), 624–632.

Hamilton, A. J. (2009). *The Scalpel and the Soul: Encounters with Surgery, the Supernatural, and the Healing Power of Hope.* Penguin Group.

Hansson, L. (1999). The Hypertension Optimal Treatment Study and The Importance of Lowering Blood Pressure. *Journal of Hypertension Supplement, 17*(1), S9–13.

Harrington, A., editor. (1999). *The Placebo Effect: An Interdisciplinary Exploration.* Harvard University Press. (Original work published February 11, 1997)

Henrich, J. (2020). *The WEIRDest People in the World: How the West Became Psychologically Peculiar and Particularly Prosperous.* Allen Lane.

Hirshberg, C. & Barasch, M. I. (1995). *Remarkable Recovery: What Extraordinary Healings Tell Us About Getting Well and Staying Well.* Riverhead Books.

Home, D.M., Pocock, S. J., Beck-Nielsen, H., Gomis, R., Hanefeld, M., Jones, N.P., Komajda, M., McMurray, J., for the RECORD Study Group. (2007). Rosiglitazone Evaluated for Cardiac Outcomes - An Interim Analysis. *New England Journal of Medicine, 357,* 28–38.

Home, D.M., (2013). Validity of Meta-Analysis in Diabetes: We Need to be Aware of Its Limitations. *Diabetes Care, 36* (10), 3361–3367.

Howard J. P., Wood, F.A., Finegold, J.A., Nowbar, A.N., Thompson, D.A., Rajkumar, C.A., Connolly, S., Cegla, J., Stride, C., Sever, P., Norton, C., Thom, S. A. M., Shun-Shin, J., Francis, D.P. (2021) Side Effect Patterns in a Crossover Trial of Statin, Placebo, and No Treatment. *Journal of the American College of Cardiology, 78* (12), 1210–1222.

Hu, F. (2003) The Mediterranean Diet and Mortality — Olive Oil and Beyond. *New England Journal of Medicine, 348,* 2595–2596.

Huang, Z., Feng, Y., Li, Y., & Lv, C. (2017). Systematic review and meta-analysis: Tai Chi for preventing falls in older adults. *BMJ Open, 7*(2). https://doi.org/10.1136/bmjopen-2016-013661

Illich, I. (2016). *Limits to Medicine. Medical Nemesis: The Expropriation of Health.* Marion Boyars Publishers. (Original work published January 1975).

International Osteoporosis Foundation. Epidemiology of Osteoporosis and Fragility Fractures. https://www.osteoporosis.foundation/facts-statistics/epidemiology-of-osteoporosis-and-fragility-fractures

Ioannidis, J. P. (2005) Contradicted and Initially Stronger Effects in Highly Cited Clinical Research, *JAMA, 294*(2), 208–218.

Ioannidis, J. P. (2005). Why Most Published Research Findings Are False. *PLOS Medicine, 2*(8). https://doi.org/10.137/journal.pmed.0020124

Ioannidis, J. P. (2013, August). How many contemporary medical practices are worse than doing nothing or doing less? *Mayo Clin Proc., 88*(10), 779–781.

Jacobs, J., Jimenez, L., Gloyd, S., Gale, J., & Crothers, D. (1994). Treatment of Acute Diarrhea with Homeopathic Medicine: A Randomized Clinical Trial in Nicaragua. *Pediatrics, 93*(5), 719–725.

Janos, J. (1947). *Janos: The Story of a Doctor.* Victor Gollancz.

John, L. K., Lowenstein, G., & Prelec, D. (2012). Measuring the Prevalence of Questionable Research Practices with Incentives for Truth Telling. *Psychological Science, 23*(5), 524–532.

Joint National Committee on Detection, Evaluation, and Treatment of High Blood Pressure. (1977). *JAMA, 237*(3), 255–261.

Kabat-Zinn, J. & Davidson, R., editors. (2011). *The Mind's Own Physician: A Scientific Dialogue with the Dalai Lama on the Healing Power of Meditation.* Presented at the Mind and Life XIII Conference in 2005. New Harbinger Publications.

Kabish, M., Ruckes, C., Seibert-Grafe, M., & Blettner, M. (2011). Randomized Controlled Trials Part 17. *Deutsches Arzteblatt International, 108*(39), 663–668. https://doi.org/10.3238/arztebl.2011.0663

Kahneman, D. (2013). *Thinking, Fast and Slow*. Farrar, Strauss, and Giroux. (Original work published 2011)

Kahneman, D., Slovic, P., & Tversky, A., editors. (1982). *Judgment Under Uncertainty; Heuristics and Biases*. Cambridge University Press.

Kam-Hansen, S., Jakubowski, M., Kelley, J. M., Kirsch, I., Hoaglin, D. C., Kaptchuk, T. J., & Burstein, R. (2014). Altered Placebo and Drug Labeling Changes the Outcome of Episodic Migraine Attacks. *Science Translational Medicine, 6*(218), 1-7. https://doi.org/ 10.1126/scitranslmed.3006175

Kandel, E. (2012). *The Age of Insight: The Quest to Understand the Unconscious in Art, Mind, and Brain, from Vienna 1900 to the Present*. Random House.

Kaptchuk, T. J., Friedlander, E., Kelley, J. M., Sanchez, M. N., Kokkotou, E., Singer, J. P., Kowalczykowski, M., Miller, F.G., Kirsch, I., Lembo, A. J. (2010). Placebos without Deception: A Randomized Controlled Trial in Irritable Bowel Syndrome. *Plos One, 5*(12), 1–7. https://doi.org/10.1371/journal.pone.0015591

Kataria, M. Laughter Yoga International. https://laughteryoga.org/#

Kearns, C. E., Schmidt, L. A., & Glantz, S. A. (2016). Sugar Industry and Coronary Heart Disease Research: A Historical Analysis of Internal Industry Documents. *JAMA Internal Medicine, 176*(11), 1680–1685.

Keys, A. B. (1980). *Seven Countries: A Multivariate Analysis of Death and Coronary Heart Disease*. Harvard University Press.

King, P., Peacock, I., & Donnelly, R. (1999). The UK Prospective Diabetes Study (UKPDS): Clinical and Therapeutic Implications for Type 2 Diabetes. *British Journal of Clinical Pharmacology, 48*(5), 643–648. https://doi.org/10.1046/j.1365-2125.1999.00092.x

Kirsch, I. & Sapirstein, G. (1998). Listening to Prozac but hearing placebo: A meta-analysis of antidepressant medication. *Prevention & Treatment, 1*(2), 1-6. https://doi.org/10.1037/1522-3736.1.1.12a

Kral, T. R. A., Schuyler, B. S., Mumford, J. A., Rosenkranz, M. A., Lutz, A., & Davidson, R. (2018). Impact of Short- and Long-term Mindfulness Meditation Training on Amygdala Reactivity to Emotional Stimuli. *Neuroimage,181*, 301–313. https://doi.org/10.1016/j.neuroimage.2018.07.013

Krasner, M. S., Epstein, R. M., Beckman, H., Suchman, A. L., Chapman, B., Mooney, C. J., & Quill, T. E., editors. (2009). Association of an Educational Program in Mindful Communication with Burnout, Empathy, and Attitudes Among Primary Care Physicians. *JAMA, 302*(12), 1284–1291.

Krishnamurti, J. & Bohm, D. (2017). *The Ending of Time: Where Philosophy and Physics Meet*. HarperOne.

Kuhn, T. (2012). *The Structure of Scientific Revolutions.* The University of Chicago Press. (Original work published 1962)

Lanier, W. L. & Rajkumar, S. V. (2013). Empiricism and Rationalism in Medicine: Can 2 Competing Philosophies Coexist to Improve the Quality of Medical Care? *Mayo Clin Proc., 88*(10), 1042–1045.

Lawrence, D.H. (1960). *Psychoanalysis and the Unconscious/Fantasia of the Unconscious.* Viking Press. (original copyright 1921)

Leibowitz, K. A., Hardebeck, E. J., Goyer, J. P., & Crum, A. J. (2018). Physician Assurance Reduces Patient Symptoms in US Adults: An Experimental Study. *Journal of General Internal Medicine 33*(12), 2051–2052. https://doi.org/10.1007/s11606-018-4627-z

Lenzer J., Hoffman, J., Furberg, C., Ioannidis, J. (2013). Ensuring the Integrity of Clinical Practice Guidelines: A Tool for Protecting Patients. *British Medical Journal, 347*, 1–10. https://doi.org/10.1136/bmj.f5535

Lerner, B. H. (2009, March 3). A Life-Changing Case for Doctors in Training. *New York Times.* www.nytimes.com/2009/03/03/health/03zion.html?ref=science

Levey, J. & Levey, M. (2014). *Living in Balance.* Divine Arts.

Levine, D. (2012). Revalidating Sherlock Holmes for a role in medical education. *Clinical Medicine, 12*(2), 146–149.

Levy, B., Pilver, C., Chung, P. H., & Slade, M. D. (2014). Subliminal Strengthening: Improving Older Individuals' Physical Function Over Time with an Implicit-Age-Stereotype Intervention. *Psychological Science, 25*, 2127-2135.

Levy, B. (1996). Improving memory in old age through implicit self-stereotyping. *Journal of Personality and Social Psychology, 71*(6), 1092-1107. https://doi.org/10.1037/0022-3514.71.6.1092

Levy, B. (2003). Mind matters: cognitive and physical effects of aging self-stereotypes. *American Journal of Gerontology, 58*(4), 203–211. https//doi.org//10.1093/geronb/58.4.

Lipid Metabolism-Atherogenesis Branch, National Heart, Lung, and Blood Institute, Bethesda, Md. (1984). The Lipid Research Clinics Coronary Primary Prevention Trial results. *JAMA, 3*(251), 365–374. https://doi.org/10.1001/jama.1984.03340270029025

Long, J. (2011). *Evidence of the Afterlife: The Science of Near-Death Experiences.* HarperCollins.

Lown, B. (1999). *The Lost Art of Healing: Practicing Compassion in Medicine.* Ballantine Books. (Original work published 1996)

Luborsky, L., Rosenthal, R., Diguer, L., Andrusyna, T. P., Berman, J. S., Levitt, J. T., Seligman, D. A., & Krause, E. D. (2002). The dodo bird verdict is alive and well—mostly. *Clinical Psychology: Science and Practice, 9*(1), 2-12. https://doi.org/10.1093/clipsy.9.1.2

Luparello, T., Lyons, H. A., Bleecker, E. R., & McFadden, E. R. (1968). Influences of suggestion on airway reactivity in asthmatic subjects. *Psychosomatic Medicine, 30*(4), 819–825.

Luparello, T. J., Leist, N., Lourie, C. H., & Sweet, P., editors. (1970). The Interaction of Psychologic Stimuli and Pharmacologic Agents on Airway Reactivity in Asthmatic Subjects. *Psychosomatic Medicine, 32*(5), 509–514.

Lutz, A., Greischar, L. L. G., Rawlings, N. B., Ricard, M., & Davidson, R. (2004). Long-term Meditators Self-Induce High-Amplitude Gamma Synchrony During Mental Practice. *PNAS, 101*(46), 16369–16373. https://doi.org/10.1073/pnas.0407401101

Maguire, E. A., Woollett, K., & Spiers, H. J. (2006). London Taxi Drivers and Bus Drivers: A Structural MRI and Neuropsychological Analysis. *Hippocampus, 16*(12), 1091–1101. https://doi.org/10.1002/hipo.20233

Mani, P. & Rohatgi, A. (2015). Niacin Therapy, HDL Cholesterol, and Cardiovascular Disease: Is the HDL Hypothesis Defunct? *Current Atherosclerosis Reports, 17*(8), 521. https://doi.org/10.1007/s11883-015-0521-x

Marchant, J. (2016). *Cure: A Journey into the Science of Mind over Body.* Crown Publishers.

Martin, S. S. & Blumenthal, R. S. (2014). Concepts and Controversies: The 2013 American College of Cardiology/American Heart Association Risk Assessment and Cholesterol Treatment Guidelines. *Annals of Internal Medicine, 5*(160), 356–358. https://doi.org/10.7326/M13-2805.

Mathie, R. T., Ramparsad, N., Legg, L. A., Clausen, J., Moss, S., Davidson, J. R. T., Messow, C., McConnachie, A. (2017, March 24). Randomised, double-blind, placebo-controlled trials of non-individualised homeopathic treatment: systematic review and meta-analysis. *Systematic Reviews, 6*(1), 63. https://doi.org/10.1186/s13643-017-0445-3

Mays, R. G., Mays S. B. (2008). The Phenomenology of the Self-Conscious Mind. *Journal of Near Death Studies, 27*(1).

McDonald, J., Janz, S. (2017, January). The Acupuncture Evidence Project. https://www.asacu.org/wp-content/uploads/2017/09/Acupuncture-Evidence-Project-The.pdf

Meador, C.K. (1992). Hex Death: Voodoo Magic or Persuasion. *Southern Medical Journal, 85*(3), 244–247.

Messer, S. B., Wampold, B. E. (2002). Let's Face Facts: Common Factors are More Potent than Specific Therapy Ingredients. *Clinical Psychology: Science and Practice, 9*(1), 21–25. https://doi.org/10.1093/clipsy.9.1.21

Meunier, P. J., Roux, C., Seeman, E., Ortolani, S., Badurski, J. E., Spector, T. D., Cannata, J., Balough, A., Lemmel, E., Pors-Nielsen, S., Rizzoli, R., Genant, H. K., & Reginster, J. (2004). The Effects of Strontium Ranelate on the Risk of Vertebral Fracture in Women with Postmenopausal Osteoporosis (SOTI trial). *New England Journal of Medicine, 350*(5), 459–468. https://doi.org/10.1056/NEJMoa022436

Michalsen, A. (2019). *The Nature Cure: A Doctor's Guide to the Science of Natural Medicine.* Viking. (Original work published 2017)

Misbin, R. I. (2007). Lessons from the Avandia Controversy. *Diabetes Care, 30*(12), 3141–3144. https://doi.org/10.2337/dc07-1908

Moerman, D. & Jonas, W. (2002). Deconstructing the Placebo Effect and Finding the Meaning Response. *Annals of Internal Medicine, 136*(6), 471–476.

Moerman, D. E. (1983, August). General Medical Effectiveness and Human Biology: Placebo Effects in the Treatment of Ulcer Disease. *Medical Anthropology Quarterly*, 1602–1606. https://doi.org/10.1525/maq.1983.14.4.02a00020

Montgomery, K. (2013). *How Doctors Think: Clinical Judgment and the Practice of Medicine.* Oxford University Press. (Original work published 2006)

Moseley, J. B., O'Malley, K., Petersen, N. J., Menke, T.J., Brody, B. A., Kuykendall, D. H., Hollingsworth, J. C., Ashton, C. A., Wray, N. (2002). A Controlled Trial of Arthroscopic Surgery for Osteoarthritis of the Knee. *New England Journal of Medicine, 347*(2), 81–88. https://doi.org/ 10.1056/NEJMoa013259

Mukherjee, S. (2015). *The Laws of Medicine: Field Notes from an Uncertain Science.* Simon and Schuster.

Murthy, V. (2020). *Together: The Healing Power of Human Connection in a Sometimes Lonely World.* HarperCollins.

National Institutes of Health. *The Framingham Heart Study: Laying the Foundation for Preventive Health Care.* www.nih.gov/sites/default/files/about-nih/impact/framingham-heart-study.pdf

National Institutes of Health. (2003). The Seventh Report of the Joint National Committee on Prevention, Detection, Evaluation, and Treatment of High Blood Pressure. https://www.nhlbi.nih.gov/files/docs/guidelines/express.pdf: *NIH Publication No.* 03-5233

Niemi, Maj-Britt. (2009, February 1). Placebo Effect: A Cure in the Mind. Scientific American. https://www.scientificamerican.com/article/placebo-effect-a-cure-in-the-mind/

Nissen, S. E. & Wolski, K. (2007). Effect of Rosiglitazone on the Risk of Myocardial Infarction and Death from Cardiovascular Causes. *New England Journal of Medicine*, 356, 2457–2471. https://doi.org/10.1056/NEJMoa072761

NMJ Contributors. (2010, May). An Evidence-based Review of Qi Gong by the Natural Standard Research Collaboration, 2(5). https://www.naturalmedicinejournal.com/journal/2010-05/evidence-based-review-qi-gong-natural-standard-research-collaboration

Nussbaum, A. M. (2016). *The Finest Traditions of My Calling: One Physician's Search for the Renewal of Medicine*. Yale University Press.

Nyoshul Khen Rinpochewell-being "Rest in Natural Great Peace." https://soundcloud.com/essentialteaching/rest-in-natural-great-peace

O'Connor, A. (2016, September 13). How the Sugar Industry Shifted Blame to Fat. www.nytimes.com/2016/09/13/well/eat/how-the-sugar-industry-shifted-blame-to-fat.html

Offit, P. (2017). *Pandora's Lab: Seven Stories of Science Gone Wrong*. National Geographic.

Olness, K. & Ader, R. (1992). Conditioning as an Adjunct in the Pharmacotherapy of Lupus Erythematosus. *Journal of Developmental and Behavioral Pediatrics*, *13*(2), 124–5.

O'Neil, C. (2016). *Weapons of Math Destruction*. Crown.

Ornish, D., Scherwitz, L. W., Billings, J. H., Brown, S. E., Gould, K. L., Merritt, T. A., Sparler, S., Armstrong, W. T., Ports, T. A., Kirkeeide, R. L., Hogeboom, C., Brand, R. J. (1998). Primary Prevention of Cardiovascular Disease with a Mediterranean Diet, *JAMA, 280*(23), 2001–2007.

Ornish D., Brown, S. E., Scherwitz, L. W., Billings, J. H., Armstrong, W. T., Ports, T. A., McLanahan, S. M., Kirkeeide, R. L., Brand, R. J., Gould, K. L. (1990). Can Lifestyle Changes Reverse Coronary Heart Disease? The Lifestyle Heart Trial. *Lancet, 336*(8708), 129–133.

Osler M.D., W. (2015). *Aequanimitas with other Addresses to Medical Students, Nurses, and Practitioners of Medicine*. Reproduction of Historical Work. Forgotten Books.

Patterson, D., Jensen, M. P., Wiechman, S. A., Sharar S. R. (2010). Virtual Reality Hypnosis for Pain Associated with Recovery from Physical Trauma. *International Journal of Clinical and Experimental Hypnosis, 58*(3), 288-300. https://doi.org/10.1080/00207141003760595

Peabody, F. (1927). The Care of the Patient. *JAMA, 88*(12), 877–882. doi:10.1001/jama.1927.02680380001001

Pincus, T. (1997). Analyzing Long-Term Outcomes of Clinical Care without Randomized Controlled Clinical Trials: The Consecutive Patient Questionnaire Database. *The Journal of Mind-Body Health, 13*(2), 3–66.

Porter, R. (1997). *The Greatest Benefit of Mankind: A Medical History of Humanity from Antiquity to the Present.* HarperCollins.

Prasad, V., Vandross, A., Toomey, C., Cheung, M., Rho, J., Quinn, S., Cifu, A. (2013). A Decade of Reversal: An Analysis of 146 Contradicted Medical Practices. *Mayo Clinic Proceedings, 88*(8), 790–798.

Prasad, V. (2013). Why Randomized Controlled Trials are Needed to Accept New Practice, 2 Medical Worldviews. *Mayo Clinic Proceedings, 88*(10), 1046–1050.

Psaty, B. & Furnberg, C. (2007). The Record on Rosiglitazone and the Risk of Myocardial Infarction. *New England Journal of Medicine, 357,* 67–69. https://doi.org/10.1056/NEJMe078116

Prentice, J. C., Conlin, P.R., Gellad W.E., Edelman, D., Lee, T.A., Pizer, S.D. (2014).

Capitalizing on Prescribing Pattern Variation to Compare Medications for Type 2 Diabetes. *Value in Health, 17*(8), 854–862. https://doi.org/10.1016/j.jval.2014.08.2674

Qin, Y., Yang, L.-H., Huang, X.-L., Chen, X.-H., & Yao, H. (2018). Efficacy and Safety of Continuous Subcutaneous Insulin Infusion vs Multiple Daily Injections on Type 1 Diabetes Children: A Meta-Analysis of Randomized Control Trials. *Journal of Clinical Research in Pediatric Endocrinology, 10*(4), 316–323. https://doi.org/10.4274/jcrpe.0053

Rankin M.D., L. (2013). *Mind Over Medicine: Scientific Proof that You Can Heal Yourself.* Hay House.

Reginster, J. Y., Seeman, E., De Verneoul, M. C., Adami, S., Compston, J., Phenekos, C., Devogelaer, J. P., Curiel, M. D., Sawicki, A., Goemaere, S., Sorensen, O. H., Felsenberg, D., Meunier, P. J. (2005). Strontium ranelate reduces the risk of nonvertebral fractures in postmenopausal women with osteoporosis: Treatment of Peripheral Osteoporosis (TROPOS) study. *Journal of Clinical Endocrinology & Metabolism, 90*(5), 2816–22. https://doi.org/10.1210/jc.2004-1774.

Reginster, J. Y., Brandi, M. L., Cannata-Andia, J., Cooper, C., Cortet, B., Feron, J. M., Genant, H., Palacios, S., Ringe, J. D., Rizzoli, R. (2015). The Position of Strontium Ranelate in Today's Management of Osteoporosis. *Osteoporosis International, 26*(6), 1667–1671.

Riggs, B. L., Hodgson, S. F., O'Fallon, W. M., Chao, E. Y. S., Wahner, H. W., Muhs, J.M., Cedel, S. L., Melon III, J. (1990). Effects of Fluoride Treatment on the Fracture Rates in Postmenopausal Women with Osteoporosis. *New England Journal of Medicine, 322*, 802–809. https://doi.org/10.1056/NEJM199003223221203

Reinhart, A. (2015). *Statistics Done Wrong: The Woefully Complete Guide*. William Pollock.

Remen, R. N. (1996). *Kitchen Table Wisdom*. Riverhead Books.

Remen, R. N. (2001). Recapturing the Soul of Medicine. Physicians Need to Reclaim Meaning in their Working Lives. *Western Journal of Medicine, 174*(1), 4–5.

Rider, M. S., Achterberg, J., Lawlis, G. F., Goven, A., Toledo, R., Butler, J. R. (1990). Effect of Immune System Imagery on Secretory IgA. *Biofeedback and Self-Regulation, 15*(4), 317–333. https://doi.org/10.1007/BF01000026.

Ridker, P. M., Danielson, E., Fonseca, A.H., Genest, J., Gotto, A., Kastelein, J. P., Koenig, W., Libby, P., Lorenzatti, A. J., MacFayden, J. G., Nordestgaard, B. G., Shepherd, J., et al for the JUPITER Study Group. (2008). Rosuvastatin to Prevent Vascular Events in Men and Women with Elevated C-Reactive Protein, *New England Journal of Medicine, 359*, 2195–2207. https://doi.org/10.1056/NEJMoa0807646

Rinpoche,S. (1993). The Tibetan Book of Living and Dying. (P. Gaffney and A. Harvey Eds)

Harper San Francisco.

Rosenstock, J., Park, G., Zimmerman, J., & US Insulin Glargine Type 1 Diabetes Investigator Group. (2000). Basal insulin glargine (HOE 901) versus NPH insulin in patients with type 1 diabetes on multiple daily insulin regimens. *Diabetes Care, 23*(8), 1137–1142. https://doi.org/10.2337/diacare.23.8.1137

Rosenthal, N. E. (2012). *Transcendence: Healing and Transformation through Transcendental Meditation*. Jeremy P. Tarcher / Penguin. (Original work published February 11, 2011)

Rosling, H. (2018). *Factfulness: Ten reasons We're Wrong About the World—and Why Things Are Better Than You Think*. Flatiron Books.

Ross, E. K. (1973). *On Death and Dying*. Macmillan and Company.

Rozanski, A., Bavishi, C., Kubzansky, L. D. (2019). Association of Optimism with Cardiovascular Events and All-Cause Mortality: A Systematic Review and Meta-Analysis. *JAMA* Network Open, 2(9), 1255. https://doi.org/10.1001/jamanetworkopen.2019.12200

Sabatine, M. S., Giugliano, R. P., Keech, A. C., Honarpur, N., Wiviott, S. D., Murphy, S. A., Kuder, J. F., Wang, H., Liu, T., Wasserman, S. M., Sever, P. S., Pedersen, T. R., FOURIER Steering Committee and Investigators. (2017). Evolocumab and Clinical Outcomes in Patients with Cardiovascular Disease. *New England Journal of Medicine,* 376 (18), 1713–1722.

Sanctis, R. W. (2021). On Being a Physician. Presented at the Harvard Medical School Class of 1958, annual lecture.

Sannes, T. S., Mansky, P. J., Chesney, M. A. (2008). The Need for Attention to Dose in Mind-Body Interventions: Lessons from Tai Chi Clinical Trials. *Journal of Alternative and Complementary Medicine,* 14(6), 645–653. https://doi.org/10.1089/acm.2007.0680

Sarrel, P. M., Katz, D. L., Njike, V. Y., & Vinante, V. (2013). The Mortality Toll of Estrogen Avoidance: An Analysis of Excess Deaths among Hysterectomized Women Aged 50 to 59 Years. *American Journal of Public Health,* 103(9), 1583–1588. https://doi.org/10.2105/AJPH.2013.301295

Schedlowski, M., Tewes, U., editors. (1999). *Psychoneuroimmunology: An Interdisciplinary Introduction.* Kluwer Academic/Plenum Publishers.

Scheutzow, M. H. (2015). Special Feature: The Women's Health Initiative (WHI) Part Four. Age Management Medicine Group E-Journal, 10(4). https://archive.agemed.org/AMMG ejournal/April2015/ScheutzowWHIWrapUpApril2015/tabid/1329/language/en-US/Default.aspx

Schlitz, M., Wiseman, R., Watt, C., & Radin, D. (2006). Of Two Minds: Sceptic-Proponent Collaboration within Parapsychology. Proceedings of the National Academy of Sciences, 97(3), 313–322. https://doi.org/10.1348/000712605X80704

Schooff, M. D. & Gupta, L. (2008). Are Long-Acting Insulin Analogues Better than Isophane Insulin? *American Family Physician,* 77(4), 447–449.

Schulz, K.F., Altman, D.G., Moher, D., for the CONSORT Group. CONSORT 2010 Statement: Updated Guidelines for Reporting Parallel Group Randomised Trials. *British Medical Journal,* 340.

Sethi, N. (2021). Antibiotics for Secondary Prevention of Coronary Heart Disease, Cochrane Database Systematic Review, 2(2):CD003610. https://doi.org/10.1002/14651858.CD003610.pub4

Siegel, B. S. (2002). *Love, Medicine & Miracles.* HarperCollins. (Original work published 1990)

Smith, A. K., White, D. B., & Arnold, R. M. (2013). Uncertainty—The Other Side of Prognosis. *New England Journal of Medicine,* 368(26), 2448–2449.

Sniderman, A. D., LaChapelle, K. J., Rachon, N. A., Furberg, C. D. (2013). The Necessity for Clinical Reasoning in the Era of Evidence-Based Medicine. Mayo Clinic Proceedings, 88(10), 1108–1114.

Song, H., Fang, F., Arnberg, F., Mataix-Clos, D., de la Cruz, L. F., Almqvist, C., Fall, K., Lichtenstein, P., Thorgeirsson, G., Valdimarsdottir, U. (2019). Stress related disorders and risk of cardiovascular disease: population based, sibling-controlled cohort study. *British Medical Journal*, 1255. https://doi.org/10.1136/bmj.l1255

Šoupal, J., Petruželková, L., Flekač, M., Pelcl, T., Matoulek, M., Dsnkova, M., Skrha, J., Svacina, S., Prazny, M. (2016). Comparison of Different Treatment Modalities for Type 1 Diabetes, Including Sensor-Augmented Insulin Regimens, in 52 Weeks of Follow-Up: A COMISAIR Study. D*iabetes Technology & Therapeutics,*18(9),532–538.

Spiegel, D., Bloom, J., Kraemer, H., & Gottheil, E. (1989). Effect of Psychosocial Treatment on Survival of Patients with Metastatic Breast Cancer. *Lancet,* 14(2), 888–891. https://doi.org/10.1016/s0140-6736(89)91551-1.

Starr, P. (2017). *The Social Transformation of American Medicine*. Basic Books. (Original work published 1982)

Steinberg, K. K., Thacker, S. B., Smith, S. J., Stroup, D. F., Zack, M. M., Flanders, D., & Berkelman, R. L. (1991). A Meta-Analysis of the Effect of Estrogen Replacement Therapy on the Risk of Breast Cancer. *JAMA*, 265(15), 1985–19903.

Stoller, J. K. (2007). Electronic Soloing: An Unintended Consequence of the Electronic Health Record. *Cleveland Clinic Journal of Medicine*, 80(7), 406–409.

Strevens, M. (2020). *The Knowledge Machine: How Irrationality Created Modern Science*. Liveright Publishing Corporation.

Strupp, H. H. & Hadley, S. W. (1979). Specific vs Nonspecific Factors in Psychotherapy: A Controlled Study of Outcomes. *Archives of General Psychiatry,* 36(10), 1125–1136.

Svanstrom, H., Pasternak, B., & Hviid, A. (2014). Use of Strontium Ranelate and Risk of Coronary Syndrome: Cohort Study. *Annals of the Rheumatic Diseases,* 73(6), 1037–1043.

Sweet V. (2012). *God's Hotel: A Doctor, a Hospital, and a Pilgrimage to the Heart of Medicine*. Riverhead Books.

Swiger, K. J., Manalac, R. J., Blumenthal, R. S., Blaha, M. J., Martin, S. S. (2013). Statins and Cognition: A Systematic Review and Meta-analysis of Short- and Long- term Cognitive Effects. Mayo Clinic Proceedings, 88(11), 1213–1221. https://doi.org/10.1016/j.mayocp.2013.07.013.

Sylvia, C. (1997). *A Change of Heart: A Memoir.* Warner Books.

Tajirian, T., Stergiopoulos, V., Strudwick, G Sequeria, L. Sanches, M. Kemp, J, Ramamoorthi, K., Zhang, T. Jankowicz, D. (2020, July). The Influence of Electronic Health Record Use on Physician Burnout: Cross-Sectional Survey. *Journal of Medical Internet Research,* 22(7). https://doi.org/10.2196/19274

Tauber, A. I. (2000). *Confessions of a Medicine Man: An Essay in Popular Philosophy.* The MIT Press. (Original work published 1999)

Thoreau, H. (1984). *Journal of Henry David Thoreau,* 1837–1861. Gibbs Smith.

Thoreau, H. (2004). *Walden.* Beacon Press.

Treatment on Morbidity and Hypertension: Results in Patients with Diastolic Pressures Averaging 115 through 129 millimeters of Mercury. (1967). *JAMA,* 1967202, 1028–1034.

Turner, J. A., Deyo, R. A., Loeser, J. D., Von Korff, M., Fordyce, W. E. (1994). The Importance of Placebo Effects in Pain Treatment and Research. *JAMA,* 271(20), 1609–1614.

Twain, M. (1907, July 5). Chapters from My Autobiography. *North American Review,* DCXVII, 466–474.

University Group Diabetes Program. (1970). A Study of the Effects of Hypoglycemic Agents on Vascular Complications in Patients with Adult-Onset Diabetes: II. Mortality Results. *Diabetes,* 19(2), 785–830.

Veterans Administration Cooperative Study Group on Antihypertensive Agents. (1970). Effects of Administration Cooperative Study Group on Antihypertensive Agents. Effects of Treatment on Morbidity in Hypertension. *JAMA,* 213(7),1143–1152.

Vickers, A. J., Brewster, S. F. (2012). PSA Velocity and Doubling Time in Diagnosis and Prognosis of Prostate Cancer. *British Journal of Medical and Surgical Urology,* 5(4), 162–168. https://doi.org/10.1016/j.bjmsu.2011.08.006

Vinkers, C. H., Lamberink, H. J., Tijdink, J.K., Heus, P., Bouter, L., Glasziou, P., Moher, D., Damen, J. A., Hooft, L., Otte, W. M. (2021) The methodological quality of 176,620 randomized controlled trials published between 1966 and 2018 reveals a positive trend but also an urgent need for improvement. *Plos Biology,* 19(4). https://doi.org/10.1371/journal.pbio.30011622021

Wachter R. (2015). *The Digital Doctor: Hope, Hype and Harm at the Dawn of Medicine's Computer Age*. McGraw Hill Education.

Wang, H., Zhu, C., Ying, Y., Luo, L., Huang, D., Luo, Z. (2018). Metformin and Berberine, Two Versatile Drugs in Treatment of Common Metabolic Diseases. *Oncotarget*, 9(11), 10135–10146.

Wright, Jr., J. T., Fine, L. J., Lackland, D. T., Ogedegbe, G., Dennison Himmelfarb, C. R. (2014). Evidence Supporting a Systolic Blood Pressure Goal of Less Than 150 mm Hg in Patients Aged 60 Years or Older: The Minority View. *Annals of Internal Medicine*, 160(7), 499–504.

Writing Group for the Women's Health Initiative Investigators. (2000). Risks and Benefits of Estrogen Plus Progestin in Healthy Postmenopausal Women. *JAMA*, 288(3), 321–333. https://doi.org/10.1001/jama.288.3.321

Yin, J., Xing, H., & Ye, J. (2008). Efficacy of Berberine in Patients with Type 2 Diabetes. *Metabolism*, 57(5), 712–717.

Youngson, R. (2012). *Time to Care*. Rebelheart Publishers.

INDEX

ABOUT THE AUTHOR

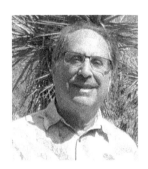

Allen Sussman was a board-certified endocrinologist in private practice for thirty-four years as well as clinical assistant professor at the University of Washington. As cofounder and president of Rainier Clinical Research Center, he was involved in hundreds of evidence-based studies and the development of ground-breaking technology for the treatment of diabetes. He also served as director of Alternative Medical Services at Valley Medical Center and participated in a Washington State Commission Taskforce to systematize standards of practice within alternative medicine.

Married to his soulmate Melanie for over thirty years, he raised with her two sons, who both became doctors. Today, Dr. Sussman lives in Seattle, Washington, where he meditates every day in a beautiful Zen garden of his own design. His interests range from Buddhist philosophy to the science of consciousness and beyond.

CPSIA information can be obtained
at www.ICGtesting.com
Printed in the USA
JSHW081944100223
37570JS00001B/28

9 781039 161788